Review of NASA's Evidence Reports on Human Health Risks

2015 LETTER REPORT

Committee to Review NASA's Evidence Reports
on Human Health Risks

Board on Health Sciences Policy

Carol E. H. Scott-Conner, Daniel R. Masys, and
Catharyn T. Liverman, *Editors*

Institute of Medicine

The National Academies of
SCIENCES · ENGINEERING · MEDICINE

THE NATIONAL ACADEMIES PRESS
Washington, DC
www.nap.edu

THE NATIONAL ACADEMIES PRESS • 500 Fifth Street, NW • Washington, DC 20001

This project was supported by Contract NNH13CK19B, Task Order NNH13CK20D, between the National Academy of Sciences and the National Aeronautics and Space Administration. Any opinions, findings, conclusions, or recommendations expressed in this publication do not necessarily reflect the views of any organization or agency that provided support for the project.

International Standard Book Number-13: 978-0-309-38061-4
International Standard Book Number-10: 0-309-38061-8
Digital Object Identifier: 10.17226/21844

Additional copies of this report available for sale from the National Academies Press, 500 Fifth Street, NW, Keck 360, Washington, DC 20001; (800) 624-6242 or (202) 334-3313; http://www.nap.edu.

Printed in the United States of America

Suggested citation: National Academies of Sciences, Engineering, and Medicine. 2016. *Review of NASA's evidence reports on human health risks: 2015 letter report.* Washington, DC: The National Academies Press. doi: 10.17226/21844.

The National Academies of
SCIENCES • ENGINEERING • MEDICINE

The **National Academy of Sciences** was established in 1863 by an Act of Congress, signed by President Lincoln, as a private, nongovernmental institution to advise the nation on issues related to science and technology. Members are elected by their peers for outstanding contributions to research. Dr. Ralph J. Cicerone is president.

The **National Academy of Engineering** was established in 1964 under the charter of the National Academy of Sciences to bring the practices of engineering to advising the nation. Members are elected by their peers for extraordinary contributions to engineering. Dr. C. D. Mote, Jr., is president.

The **National Academy of Medicine** (formerly the Institute of Medicine) was established in 1970 under the charter of the National Academy of Sciences to advise the nation on medical and health issues. Members are elected by their peers for distinguished contributions to medicine and health. Dr. Victor J. Dzau is president.

The three Academies work together as the **National Academies of Sciences, Engineering, and Medicine** to provide independent, objective analysis and advice to the nation and conduct other activities to solve complex problems and inform public policy decisions. The Academies also encourage education and research, recognize outstanding contributions to knowledge, and increase public understanding in matters of science, engineering, and medicine.

Learn more about the National Academies of Sciences, Engineering, and Medicine at **www.national-academies.org**.

COMMITTEE TO REVIEW NASA'S EVIDENCE REPORTS ON HUMAN HEALTH RISKS

CAROL E. H. SCOTT-CONNER (*Chair*), University of Iowa Carver College of Medicine, Iowa City
DANIEL R. MASYS (*Vice Chair*), University of Washington, Seattle
SUSAN A. BLOOMFIELD, Texas A&M University, College Station
C. PATRICK DUNNE, Dunne Solutions, Framingham, MA
BRAD HOLSCHUH, University of Minnesota, Twin Cities
MICHAEL J. JOYNER, Mayo Clinic, Rochester, MN
JAMES A. PAWELCZYK, Pennsylvania State University, University Park
K. P. SANDEEP, North Carolina State University, Raleigh
ROBERT L. SATCHER, JR., University of Texas, Houston
JACK STUSTER, Anacapa Sciences, Santa Barbara, CA
SCOTT TRAPPE, Ball State University, Muncie, IN
PETER D. WAGNER, University of California, San Diego
GAYLE E. WOLOSCHAK, Northwestern University Feinberg School of Medicine, Chicago, IL
LAURENCE R. YOUNG, Massachusetts Institute of Technology, Cambridge

IOM Staff

CATHARYN T. LIVERMAN, Study Director
CLAIRE F. GIAMMARIA, Research Associate
JUDITH L. ESTEP, Program Associate
SOPHIE YANG, Research Assistant
ANDREW M. POPE, Director, Board on Health Sciences Policy

Reviewers

This report has been reviewed in draft form by individuals chosen for their diverse perspectives and technical expertise. The purpose of this independent review is to provide candid and critical comments that will assist the institution in making its published report as sound as possible and to ensure that the report meets institutional standards for objectivity, evidence, and responsiveness to the study charge. The review comments and draft manuscript remain confidential to protect the integrity of the deliberative process. We wish to thank the following individuals for their review of this report:

ELDON W. ASKEW, University of Utah
DENNIS R. HELDMAN, The Ohio State University
SUSAN R. HOPKINS, University of California, San Diego
DAVID KIRSCH, Duke University Medical Center
JOANNE LUPTON, Texas A&M University
NEAL W. POLLOCK, Duke University Medical Center
FRANK A. SLOAN, Duke University
JOHN B. WEST, University of California, San Diego

Although reviewers listed above have provided many constructive comments and suggestions, they did not see the final draft of the report before its release. The review of this report was overseen by **GLORIA LEON,** University of Minnesota, who served as the coordinator. She was responsible for making certain that an independent examination of this report was carried out in accordance with institutional procedures and that all review comments were carefully considered. Responsibility for the final content of this report rests entirely with the authoring committee and the institution.

Contents

APPENDIXES

The National Academies of
SCIENCES · ENGINEERING · MEDICINE

INSTITUTE OF MEDICINE
Board on Health Sciences and Policy

December 28, 2015

Mark Shelhamer, Ph.D.
Lyndon B. Johnson Space Center
2101 NASA Parkway
Houston, TX 77058

Dear Dr. Shelhamer:

The Institute of Medicine (IOM), at the request of the National Aeronautics and Space Administration (NASA) and with guidance from the IOM's Standing Committee on Aerospace Medicine and the Medicine of Extreme Environments (CAMMEE), has established the Committee to Review NASA's Evidence Reports on Human Health Risks. This letter report is the third in a series of five reports (IOM, 2014, 2015). The committee will provide an independent review of the more than 30 evidence reports that NASA has compiled on human health risks for long-duration and exploration spaceflights. This 2015 letter report builds on the work of the 2008 IOM report and examines seven evidence reports:

1. *Risk of Impaired Performance Due to Reduced Muscle Mass, Strength, and Endurance* (Ploutz-Snyder et al., 2015),
2. *Risk of Reduced Physical Performance Capabilities Due to Reduced Aerobic Activity* (Downs et al., 2015),
3. *Risk of Orthostatic Intolerance During Re-exposure to Gravity* (Stenger et al., 2015),
4. *Risk of Injury and Compromised Performance Due to Extravehicular Activity (EVA) Operations* (Chappell et al., 2015),
5. *Risk of Decompression Sickness* (Conkin et al., 2013),
6. *Risk of Performance Decrement and Crew Illness Due to an Inadequate Food System* (Perchonok et al., 2012), and
7. *Risk Factor of Inadequate Nutrition* (Smith et al., 2015).

COMMITTEE'S TASK AND OVERARCHING ISSUES

To review the seven NASA evidence reports, the IOM assembled a 14-member committee with expertise in aerospace medicine, occupational health, radiation medicine, human performance, internal medicine, physiology and exercise science, respiratory health, behavioral health, food sciences and nutrition, human factors engineering, materials sciences, and biomedical informatics. Committee biographical sketches are included in Appendix B.

The committee's task, detailed in Box 1, was to review each evidence report in response to nine specific questions. In summary, this report examines the quality of the evidence, analysis, and overall construction of each report; identifies existing gaps in report content; and provides suggestions for additional sources of expert input. This report also builds on the 2008 IOM report *Review of NASA's Human Research Program Evidence Books: A Letter Report*, which assessed the process for developing NASA's evidence reports and provided an initial and brief review of NASA's original evidence report.[1]

The committee approached its task by analyzing each evidence report's overall quality, which included readability; internal consistency; the source and breadth of cited evidence; identification of existing knowledge and research gaps; authorship expertise; and, if applicable, response to recommendations from the IOM letter report previously described.

It is difficult to characterize and compare the quality of evidence cited in individual evidence reports. In the 2008 letter report, the IOM urged NASA to "require authors to use categories of evidence in future versions of the evidence books, while recognizing that experience with the explicit categorization of evidence may be refined over time, particularly regarding the categories used" (IOM, 2008, p. 12). NASA encourages evidence report authors "to label evidence according to the 'NASA Categories of Evidence'" (NASA, 2013a).[2] Authors of NASA evidence reports should be encouraged to adhere to standard guidelines for systematic reviews (IOM, 2011; Huguet et al., 2013; Wallace et al., 2013).

---

[1]The original evidence book was "a collection of evidence reports created from the information presented verbally and discussed within the NASA HRP [Human Research Program] in 2006" (NASA, 2013a).

[2]NASA has identified three categories of evidence that could be included in each evidence report, including data from controlled experiments, observational studies, and expert opinion (NASA, 2013a).

Furthermore, as noted in prior IOM letter reports (IOM, 2014, 2015), substantial variability exists in the formatting, internal consistency, and completeness of the references among individual evidence reports, making it difficult to compare cited evidence for related human health risks. NASA is encouraged to select a preferred citation format for all evidence reports and to require all writing teams to use that format.

BOX 1
Review of NASA's Evidence Reports on Human Health Risks
Statement of Task

NASA has requested a study from the Institute of Medicine (IOM) to provide an independent review of more than 30 evidence reports on human health risks for long duration and exploration spaceflight. The evidence reports, which are publicly available, are categorized into five broad categories: (1) behavioral health and performance; (2) human health countermeasures (with a focus on bone metabolism and orthopedics, nutrition, immunology, and cardiac and pulmonary physiology); (3) radiation; (4) human factors issues; and (5) exploration medical capabilities. The reports are revised on an ongoing basis to incorporate new scientific information. In conducting this study, an IOM ad hoc committee will build on the 2008 IOM report *Review of NASA's Human Research Program Evidence Books*. That report provided an assessment of the process used for developing the evidence reports and provided an initial review of the evidence reports that had been completed at that time.

Each year, NASA staff will identify a set of evidence reports for committee review. Over the course of the study all evidence reports will be reviewed. The committee will hold an annual scientific workshop to receive input on the evidence reports it is reviewing that year and an update on the recent literature. The committee will issue an annual letter report that addresses the following questions relevant to each evidence report:

1. Does the evidence report provide sufficient evidence, as well as sufficient risk context, that the risk is of concern for long-term space missions?
2. Does the evidence report make the case for the research gaps presented?
3. Are there any additional gaps in knowledge or areas of fundamental research that should be considered to enhance the basic understanding of this specific risk?
4. Does the evidence report address relevant interactions among risks?
5. Is input from additional disciplines needed?
6. Is the breadth of the cited literature sufficient?

7. What is the overall readability and quality?
8. Is the expertise of the authors sufficient to fully cover the scope of the given risk?
9. Has the evidence report addressed previous recommendations made by the IOM in the 2008 letter report?

In addition to analyzing the content of individual letter reports, the committee also gathered evidence from existing literature and relevant experts in the field. The committee held two conference call meetings and one in-person meeting, with the latter held in conjunction with a public workshop (see Appendix A). At the workshop, the committee invited individuals with expertise related to at least one of the seven evidence reports to analyze NASA's evidence reports and engage in discussions with the committee, focusing on the following questions:

- How well is the risk understood?
- What, if any, are the major sources of disagreement in the literature pertaining to this risk?
- What are the main gaps in knowledge or fundamental research about the risk?
- What is known about interactions between the risk and other risks identified in NASA's evidence reports?

This report follows the format of the prior IOM letter reports, which includes the committee's responses to each of the questions listed in its statement of task for each of the seven evidence reports. Although no formal recommendations are included in this report, the committee's observations are intended to inform and improve NASA's ongoing efforts to update the content of individual evidence reports.

THE NASA HUMAN RESEARCH ROADMAP

The evidence reports reviewed in this IOM report are part of a larger roadmap process developed and under implementation by NASA's Human Research Program (HRP). The goals of the HRP are to "provide human health and performance countermeasures, knowledge, technologies, and tools to enable safe, reliable, and productive human space exploration" (NASA, 2014a). As outlined in Figure 1, the evidence reports

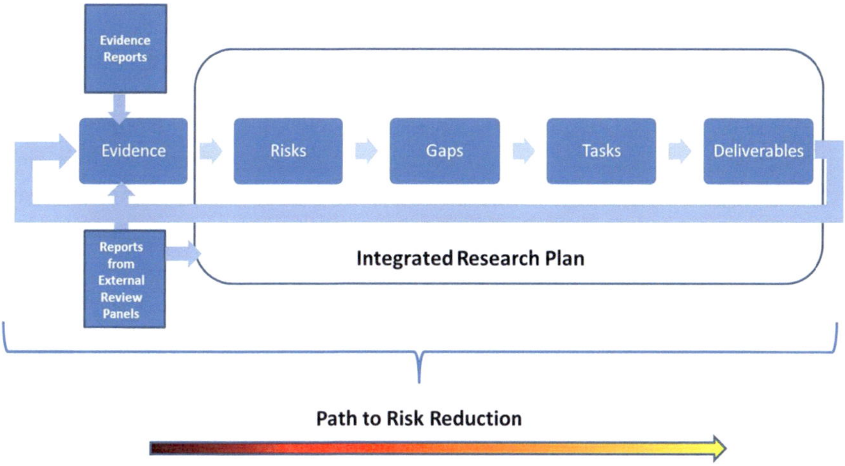

FIGURE 1 NASA's human research roadmap.
SOURCE: Adapted from NASA, 2014a.

are the first part of the roadmap, which is followed by clarifying the risks, specifying the research gaps to address those risks, implementing research tasks, and obtaining deliverables. These steps are then assessed to ascertain progress in preventing or mitigating the risk to astronaut health. NASA updates its progress on risk reduction for four design reference missions: (1) 12-month mission on the International Space Station (ISS); (2) lunar (outpost) mission; (3) deep space journey mission (e.g., near Earth asteroid); and (4) planetary mission (e.g., Mars) by identifying the extent to which there is evidence that the plans for that mission will meet existing crew health standards or that countermeasures exist to control the risk (NASA, 2013b).

RISK OF IMPAIRED PERFORMANCE DUE TO REDUCED MUSCLE MASS, STRENGTH, AND ENDURANCE

Human spaceflight missions have evolved over the past 50 years from short duration missions lasting only minutes to current missions lasting up to 1 year on the ISS. The evidence report *Risk of Impaired Performance Due to Reduced Muscle Mass, Strength, and Endurance* (Ploutz-Snyder et al., 2015) provides a substantive overview of the breadth of evidence regarding the risks related to skeletal muscle health and documents the wealth of data that have been obtained through prior spaceflights as well as through human ground-based studies and animal experiments. As noted in the evidence report, it has become apparent that as mission duration progresses, skeletal muscle health and performance deficits occur. These skeletal muscle deficits pose potentially serious risk to crewmembers on multiple levels. In addition to documenting the risk, the evidence report also highlights historical and current perspectives of exercise countermeasure development, the evolution of exercise hardware, and the complexities associated with minimizing the reductions in skeletal muscle mass and resulting decrements in function with spaceflight. The authors rely on the scientific literature and NASA technical reports to provide a comprehensive document. The committee's responses to the key review questions are summarized below.

Does the Evidence Report Provide Sufficient Evidence, as Well as Sufficient Risk Context, That the Risk Is of Concern for Long-Term Space Missions?

The evidence report provides an excellent summary of manned spaceflight from the early missions to current 6-month stays on the ISS. Numerous aspects of skeletal muscle health and its intersection with exercise programs and hardware (i.e., exercise devices) are presented. Likewise, animal data and myocellular findings related to the mechanistic aspect of skeletal muscle in microgravity are also presented. Several knowledge gaps are identified, and numerous suggestions for future research are presented.

The report would be improved by providing a more detailed description of the exercise dosing/titration models used to mitigate skeletal muscle loss with microgravity. As highlighted by the author team, there has been excellent progress in the countermeasure program for skeletal muscle in the past 20 years from ground analogs, including bed rest and animal studies using unilateral lower-limb suspension to space shuttle and ISS observations that clearly show that high-intensity exercise is beneficial. However, details on the exercise protocol progression (sets, reps, timing, and dosing of aerobic, anaerobic, and resistance exercise) should be more thoroughly profiled to help guide the exercise prescription into the future.

Does the Evidence Report Make the Case for the Research Gaps Presented?

Several gaps are identified with excellent justification from relevant tasks for successful and safe space travel with varied mission objectives. Furthermore, scientifically based evidence is presented where appropriate to further highlight the potential health risks associated with spaceflight.

Figure 11 in the evidence report (Figure 2 below) highlights the large individual variability in muscle strength changes with long-duration stays on the ISS and stands out as an example of the challenges with skeletal muscle health with spaceflight. Interestingly, the variability presented is well outside the range observed in numerous human ground-based analog studies (i.e., bed rest). This is most likely a result of varied approaches to the exercise program, hardware, preflight fitness levels of the crew, as well as other confounding factors of working in space and the genotypic and phenotypic variability between crewmembers.

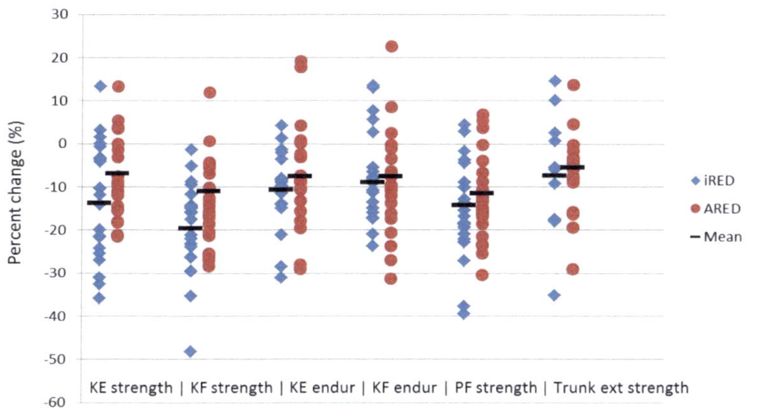

Figure 11. Post-flight changes (%) in isokinetic leg and trunk strength for long-duration ISS crewmembers using iRED and ARED during their flight.

FIGURE 2 Post-flight changes (percent change) in isokinetic leg and trunk strength for long-duration ISS crewmembers using iRED (interim Resistive Exercise Device) and ARED (Advanced Resistive Exercise Device) during their flight.
NOTE: KE = knee extensor, KF = knee flexor, PF (not defined).
SOURCE: Ploutz-Snyder et al., 2015.

Are There Any Additional Gaps in Knowledge or Areas of Fundamental Research That Should Be Considered to Enhance the Basic Understanding of This Specific Risk?

Additional knowledge gaps that relate to the skeletal muscle health challenges associated with long-duration space travel could be added, including the following:

- Further define skeletal muscle-specific tasks and the performance parameters (muscle groups used, strength, power, and duration) necessary to perform these tasks. This is paramount for understanding the muscle performance necessary to execute mission-specific objectives and emergency contingencies. This needs to be defined both for steady-state spaceflight experiences and for transition states to other planets. Understanding the task requirements is critical to defining minimum fitness for duty standards, which also serve as a measure of countermeasure efficacy.
- Further research is needed to identify the proper balance of aerobic and resistance exercise best suited to protect skeletal muscle health during spaceflight, especially in light of Figure 11 of the evidence report that shows the extensive differences in individual variability. To date, the exercise prescription remains incomplete, and more scientific data at the whole body and cell level are needed to further elucidate the best exercise paradigm. Skeletal muscle biology is complex with varied integrated responses in the minutes, hours, and days following an exercise stimulus. The muscle biology response also varies depending on the exercise mode (aerobic versus resistance) and the timing relative to successive exercise bouts. These concepts need to be more thoroughly understood in order to develop a complete exercise countermeasure for skeletal muscle health that will likely affect other physiological and organ systems. Further, human physiology and the response to exercise vary based on genotype, so countermeasures may need to be varied on an individual basis.
- A practical method is needed to monitor, at the individual astronaut level, performance characteristics of important muscle groups and could include muscle imaging (for size and thickness). This will help guide individual exercise prescriptions during adaption to microgravity.

- Breaks from exercise and variation in the exercise regimen (termed periodization) are likely to be required during a long-duration mission to Mars. Breaks may also be required during recovery from injury or to prevent overtraining, and rehabilitation plans are needed to account for time off from the exercise-training program that may occur from injury or illness. Little is known about periodic time off during the training routine in a microgravity environment and how this will affect skeletal muscle health and other physiological systems.
- The nutritional interface with skeletal muscle adaptation needs attention and could provide new strategic opportunities to enhance the skeletal muscle response to exercise. It is likely that the timing (before, during, and after exercise) of carbohydrate and protein intake could positively enhance the biological response to exercise in the space environment. Numerous examples in the sport science literature support this concept and could be used as initial guidance. However, more work on the unique interface of skeletal muscle in a microgravity environment (real and simulated) with exercise and nutrition is an area that warrants further exploration and could be a crosscutting platform with various metabolic aspects of skeletal muscle (i.e., substrate flux, microcirculation/blood flow) to enhance/impact the exercise program.
- The discussion on hormone interaction with skeletal muscle should be expanded beyond insulin. There are likely key regulatory aspects of cortisol, androgens, estrogen, and myokines that would affect the net protein balance of skeletal muscle. Evidence is emerging that skeletal muscle acts as a secretory organ, with myokines being responsive to exercise and mediators of inflammation, as well as evidence of crosstalk with other organ systems (Pedersen and Febbraio, 2012; Pratesi et al., 2013). Circadian rhythm(s) and their influence on hormonal balance and muscle physiology and performance should be further explored. As a result, this area has the potential to impact health beyond skeletal muscle and would be crosscutting for other biological systems (i.e., systems biology).
- The effect of pharmaceuticals on muscle biology and exercise response warrants investigation. Both over-the-counter (i.e., non-steroidal anti-inflammatory drugs) and prescription (i.e., statins) are known to impact muscle physiology and exercise response

(Trappe et al., 2002, 2011). Various medications used during a mission could potentially interact with skeletal muscle biology in such a way as to influence the anabolic and catabolic state of the muscle and the subsequent response to exercise.

- Attention to potential sex differences in skeletal muscle adaptation to microgravity and the response to exercise needs to be strongly considered. This was recommended in the 2008 IOM report and does not appear to have been addressed. Growing evidence in the literature shows that sex differences are apparent in the biological response to exercise and various populations groups (Hunter, 2014; Ploutz-Snyder et al., 2014).
- Impact of preflight fitness and training status on the rate and extent of muscle function loss is important to define, especially as it relates to countermeasure development. Moreover, preflight fitness and training status intersect with task-specific demands and physiological reserve, which may be critical in gravitational transition states and emergency situations.

Does the Evidence Report Address Relevant Interactions Among Risks?

The report does an excellent job discussing the interactions among the risks listed in the evidence report. However, as highlighted above, additional interactions with skeletal muscle related to nutrition, hormones/myokines, pharmacokinetics, disrupted circadian rhythms, sex, and defining minimum muscle strength and power requirements for mission tasks (e.g., EVAs) should be explored and discussions of potential interactions should be added to the relevant evidence reports. The committee also noted the potential impact of exercise devices on various physiological systems (i.e., integrative biology). In particular, the potential influence of the relatively new Advanced Resistance Exercise Device (ARED) on intraocular pressure is of recent research interest (IOM, 2014). The committee expressed interest in energy balance as it relates to exercise (i.e., oxygen consumption), nutrient intake, and storage of enough food supplies to support a mission. Lastly, exercise as a mood enhancer during extended space missions was discussed and would be interactive with various psychological parameters.

What Is the Overall Readability and Quality?

The report was well written and organized to provide a high-quality document that was easy to follow and comprehend.

Is the Breadth of the Cited Literature Sufficient?

For the topics directly covered in this report the cited references were comprehensive. However, it is likely the narrative and supporting references will need to be expanded to adequately address the newly identified knowledge gaps.

Is the Expertise of the Authors Sufficient to Fully Cover the Scope of the Given Risk? Is Input from Additional Disciplines Needed?

The expertise of the author team is excellent, although additional perspectives may be beneficial to expand the knowledge to include other disciplines that are emerging (i.e., myokines) or intersect with other physiological systems (i.e., nutrition) that will address the additional knowledge gaps identified.

There are several emerging areas resulting in additional knowledge gaps involving skeletal muscle health that intersect with other disciplines (i.e., nutrition, microcirculation, hormone biology, drug interactions) that will most likely require additional input from experts in these areas for future iterations of the evidence report. These crosscutting areas further highlight the complex and integrated nature of these systems.

Has the Evidence Report Addressed Previous Recommendations Made by the IOM in the 2008 Letter Report?

The evidence report addressed several of the recommendations of the previous report to provide a more comprehensive discussion related to human control subjects and a more detailed overview of the progression in exercise countermeasures over the past 50 years. The 2008 report recommended that sex-related issues for skeletal muscle health be discussed in the context of spaceflight. However, this is still lacking in the current evidence report. Partially addressed is the effectiveness of various exercise modalities. This was primarily due to the limited published data available in this area, and it is recommended that this continue to evolve with subsequent reports.

RISK OF REDUCED PHYSICAL PERFORMANCE CAPABILITIES DUE TO REDUCED AEROBIC CAPACITY

A solid base of evidence is available on the nature of the aerobic deconditioning that occurs with spaceflight, as well as on the physiological mechanisms that underpin this deconditioning, ground-based analogs of reduced gravity, and exercise countermeasures (e.g., Convertino et al., 2010; Lee et al., 2010). Evidence has also been published on the interactions between these factors and thermoregulation and orthostatic intolerance (Guinet et al., 2009; Mekjavic et al., 2012). Additionally, much of this evidence can be framed in the context of routine performance demands in space and also more extreme challenges such as EVAs. The evidence report *Risk of Reduced Physical Performance Capabilities Due to Reduced Aerobic Capacity* (Downs et al., 2015) provides an overview highlighting historical and current perspectives on exercise countermeasure development. The report draws primarily on observational and experimental data collected during and after spaceflight along with human ground-based analog studies (i.e., bed rest). The authors rely on the scientific literature and NASA technical reports to provide a comprehensive document. The committee's responses to the key review questions are summarized below.

Does the Evidence Report Provide Sufficient Evidence, as Well as Sufficient Risk Context, That the Risk Is of Concern for Long-Term Space Missions?

The evidence report provides an excellent summary of issues related to maintenance of maximal aerobic capacity during manned spaceflights from the early missions to current 6-month stays on the ISS. However, aerobic capacity (VO_2 max), while often used as a metric of maximal exercise ability, does not closely reflect the capacity to perform a submaximal task, particularly if effort is required for more than a short time. Therefore, this evidence report needs to be focused more directly on the development, maintenance, and mitigation of task-specific physiological capacity before and during any envisioned mission. The report is focused largely on changes in VO_2 max or peak work capacity, how it is affected by spaceflight duration, and how these changes are affected by individual differences in astronauts. For example, the report describes the effects of baseline fitness and the role of exercise intensity as potential modifiers of the fall in VO_2 max during spaceflight. The key roles of changes in stroke volume and plasma/blood volume are highlighted throughout the report. Several knowledge gaps are identified and numerous suggestions for future research presented.

The report would be strengthened by providing additional information on arm-specific aerobic exercise capacity in response to spaceflight and/or bed rest. The rationale is that certain high stress EVA tasks have a major upper-body component.

Given the work on intense aerobic training followed by reduced training intensity, frequency, or duration published primarily during the 1980s, the committee found it surprising that more information on related topics is not available (e.g., Hickson et al., 1982, 1984, 1985). To the extent that information is available on these topics it should be added to the evidence report.

Does the Evidence Report Make the Case for the Research Gaps Presented?

Several gaps were identified with excellent justification from relevant tasks for successful and safe space travel with varied mission objectives. Furthermore, scientifically based evidence was presented to further highlight the potential health risks associated with spaceflight. Several of the gaps focused on the need to better understand the peak aerobic physiological stresses (intensity and duration) on crews and how fitness standards and interventions could be most efficiently designed to meet these potential stresses. However, these stressors are likely to have at least some intermittent exercise elements and also require muscular strength and coordination. This information should be integrated with the Muscle Mass evidence report (Ploutz-Snyder et al., 2015) discussed above so a comprehensive strategy can be developed. The need to integrate the physiology with exercise hardware is also key, especially if there is to be greater focus on upper-body aerobic performance.

Are There Any Additional Gaps in Knowledge or Areas of Fundamental Research That Should Be Considered to Enhance the Basic Understanding of This Specific Risk?

The knowledge gaps presented at the end of the report are comprehensive. The following areas are highlighted as areas where additional emphasis might be useful:

- Further define tasks and the aerobic capabilities necessary to perform these tasks for spaceflight experiences and transition states to other planets. This is paramount for understanding the physiological capacity necessary to execute mission-specific objectives and emergency contingencies.
- Improved understanding of upper-body aerobic capacity and related countermeasures, because many tasks require substantial upper-body efforts.
- Expanding the evidence base for the concept that occasional minimal-duration, high-intensity exercise bouts might be highly protective against declines in VO_2 max and also reduce the need for prolonged exercise training sessions.
- Better understanding of emerging evidence about blood-flow-restricted exercise as a way to increase the efficacy of the exercise training stimulus.
- The potential usefulness of occasional training with intentional thermal stress to both increase plasma volume and maintain aerobic capacity.
- The need to integrate the aerobic exercise countermeasure standards with:
    - Skeletal muscle standards.
    - Nutrition planning relevant to voluntary exercise and food needs. Such planning should include both the minimal exercise needed to maintain fitness, and some additional "voluntary" exercise for recreation and for mood elevation.
    - Integration of the fitness standards with performance requirements and consideration of these requirements in the context of technology or other ergonomic approaches that might limit these demands.
- The exploitation of inter-individual physiological capacity to match individual crewmember physiology to the tasks they are assigned.

In agreement with the Muscle Mass report (Ploutz-Snyder et al., 2015) described above, there is a need to emphasize the following issues:

- The exercise dose–response relationship needs further research to identify the proper balance of aerobic and resistance exercise best suited to protect both aerobic capacity and skeletal muscle health during spaceflight. To date, the exercise prescription remains incomplete and more scientific data at the whole body and cell level are needed to further elucidate the best exercise paradigm.
- A simple way to monitor individual astronaut aerobic as well as skeletal muscle strength during mission needs to be developed. In a manner similar to that described for the previous report, this would allow modification of the individual exercise prescription as needed.
- Improved understanding is needed of the effect of nutritional intake and its timing relative to exercise on the physiological response to exercise.
- Preflight fitness and training status, including upper-body exercise capacity, should be addressed as these variables have the likelihood to affect the adaptive response to microgravity and subsequent countermeasures to combat the loss of aerobic capacity. Moreover, pre-flight fitness and training status intersect with task-specific demands and physiological reserve, which may be critical in gravitational transition states and emergency situations.

Does the Evidence Report Address Relevant Interactions Among Risks?

The report does an excellent job discussing the interactions among the risks listed in the evidence report, in particular the interactions between aerobic deconditioning and orthostatic intolerance. Discussion of interactions with the performance issues raised in the EVA evidence report (Chappell et al., 2015) could be added.

What Is the Overall Readability and Quality?

The report was well written and organized to provide a high-quality document that was easy to follow and comprehend.

Is the Breadth of the Cited Literature Sufficient?

For the topics directly covered in this report the cited references were comprehensive. However, it is likely the narrative and supporting references will need to be expanded to adequately address the newly identified knowledge gaps. Key areas to consider include older and more recent data on short-duration, high-intensity intervals as a way to protect aerobic capacity and also emerging ideas about blood flow restriction during training as a method to enhance peripheral adaptations to exercise.

Is the Expertise of the Authors Sufficient to Fully Cover the Scope of the Given Risk? Is Input from Additional Disciplines Needed?

The expertise of the author team is quite good, although additional perspectives as outlined above might be helpful. There are several emerging areas resulting in additional knowledge gaps. As noted above, the aerobic exercise standards, performance demands, and training interventions need ongoing integration with the skeletal muscle and nutrition evidence base. All of these need to be integrated with the physiological demands of anticipated and emergency tasks. They also need to be integrated with many logistical and ergonomic issues from areas such as nutrition, sleep, suit design, and psychology.

Has the Evidence Report Addressed Previous Recommendations Made by the IOM in the 2008 Letter Report?

The evidence report addressed several of the recommendations of the previous report to provide a more comprehensive discussion related to human control subjects and a more detailed overview of the progression in exercise countermeasures over the past 50 years. The 2008 report recommended the following:

> The gaps should include preflight fitness requirements for cardiovascular capacity relating to prolonged space travel. Gender should also be considered as a potential gap. Although gender-related data are limited, it does point to a potential issue. Gaps 4 and 6 should include cardiac and skeletal muscle mass as potentially important contributors to cardiovascular performance. (p. 55)

As noted above, gaps identical to or directly related to this gap from 2008 persist.

RISK OF ORTHOSTATIC INTOLERANCE DURING RE-EXPOSURE TO GRAVITY

The problem of orthostatic intolerance—an inability to adequately regulate blood pressure after spaceflight when body posture is aligned with a substantial positive gravity gradient—has been recognized since the final Mercury mission (34-hours duration). The evidence report *Risk of Orthostatic Intolerance During Re-Exposure to Gravity* (Stenger et al., 2015) provides an overview of the solid base of evidence that exists on the nature of the problem including documenting the relevant experiences from the Shuttle, Mir, and ISS eras. On Earth, orthostatic hypotension can have many causes. It affects approximately 5 percent of patients under 50 years of age, increasing as a function of age to 30 percent of those over 70 years of age (Ricci et al., 2015). Similarly, there is a good understanding of the physiological mechanisms that underpin it and the interactions with other stresses, including thermal stress, nutrition/hydration, and physical (in)activity.

Orthostatic intolerance is not as much a problem during the orbital or cruise phases of spaceflight as it is during launch, landing, and egress (Stenger et al., 2015). However, it should be noted that orthostatic intolerance is most predictably evoked by quiescent standing without engagement of the muscle pump at times of changing from less to more gravitational stress. Orthostatic intolerance is thus unlikely to occur during sustained microgravity; after adjustment (perhaps hours to days) to a new gravitational field greater than that to which the astronaut has been exposed; and during the transient phase of landing and spacecraft egress after flight, when active muscular effort is usually required (Stenger et al., 2015).

This evidence report draws on observational and experimental data collected during and after spaceflight along with human ground-based analog studies (e.g., hypovolemia and bed rest). The authors rely on the scientific literature and NASA technical reports to provide an evidence report that is comprehensive and well written.

Does the Evidence Report Provide Sufficient Evidence, as Well as Sufficient Risk Context, That the Risk Is of Concern for Long-Term Space Missions?

The evidence report summarizes the incidence of orthostatic intolerance well, highlighting the observation that the incidence of orthostatic intolerance is directly related to the duration of exposure to microgravity during spaceflight. The evidence report posits sex-specific differences in orthostatic intolerance. As further discussed below, a critical gap identified in the evidence report concerns the unknowns regarding how exploration-duration flights (greater than 1 year) will affect orthostatic intolerance and cardiovascular regulation. Whether extremely long voyages, such as to Mars, increase the risk after landing on a planet with substantially less gravity than on Earth is of course unknown. The evidence report also makes the case that orthostatic intolerance recovers rapidly following return to 1G, but there is a fundamental lack of evidence regarding landing in or return from fractional G environments. The evidence report provides an extensive discussion of the multifactorial etiology of orthostatic intolerance, including fluid redistribution, hypovolemia, cardiac/vascular atrophy, and autonomic dysregulation. Each of these factors can induce orthostatic intolerance.

Does the Evidence Report Make the Case for the Research Gaps Presented?

The evidence report provides a substantive review of the mechanisms that contribute to orthostatic intolerance. The gaps focus appropriately on orthostatic intolerance in lunar and Mars gravitational fields, which can be mimicked using head-up tilt at approximately +10° and +22°, respectively. It is not known if these gradients are sufficient to evoke orthostatic intolerance, and further, if prolonged exposure to partial gravity environments will evoke intolerance when shorter exposures would not.

A considerable section of the evidence report reviews modeling approaches to predict susceptibility to orthostatic intolerance. Several dynamic models are reviewed, which can be used to simulate compensatory responses to standing and changes comparable to short-term exposures to a free fall environment. The evidence report authors appropriately describe a lack of rigorous verification, validation, and uncertain quantification procedures for these models. Structural equation modeling has provided some utility and could help fill this gap (Wallace et al., 2010).

The evidence report includes a thorough discussion of potential countermeasures to ameliorate orthostatic intolerance. Five categories of countermeasures are featured: fluid loading, artificial gravity, lower-body negative pressure during microgravity, pharmacotherapy, and compression garments during transition stages. Overall, this section is well organized and the literature cited in each area is appropriate, including a mix of fundamental and operational research.

Are There Any Additional Gaps in Knowledge or Areas of Fundamental Research That Should Be Considered to Enhance the Basic Understanding of This Specific Risk?

The committee has identified additional areas to be considered in future iterations of this evidence report:

- Fractional gravity is addressed appropriately, but available data are relatively incomplete. The orthostatic stress imposed by lunar or Martian gravity could be sufficiently large to constitute a risk when transitioning from prolonged flights in zero-G gravity. Alternatively, in expedition-class missions chronic exposure to these fields could have a protective effect against cardiovascular deconditioning.
- Orthostatic intolerance can be evoked in any human being if the imposed orthostatic stress is of sufficient magnitude and duration. The extent to which this affects operational capabilities has not been established. The evidence report provides no reports of orthostatic events during ascent or re-entry phases of spaceflight.
- There is a well-established interaction between thermal stress and orthostatic intolerance, associated with a displacement of a portion of circulating blood volume to the compliant cutaneous vascular bed. This interaction could occur during launch and entry if suit cooling is inadequate.
- Individual susceptibility to and variability in severity of orthostatic intolerance are not well defined.
- Adrenergic receptor biology and excitation–contraction coupling in vascular smooth muscle have not been included in the review. Both hind-limb suspension models and spaceflight have revealed substantial changes that could impair sympathetic transduction—

the coupling of sympathetic activity to a vascular smooth muscle response. Several coupled elements determine the response, including norepinephrine release in response to depolarization, sensitivity to released norepinephrine, activation of adrenergic signaling cascades, and smooth muscle contraction. A number of countermeasures to improve orthostatic intolerance are discussed in the review but their comparative effectiveness needs to be analyzed.

- The efficacy of combination countermeasure treatment is not particularly well developed, which is reflective of the state of the literature at this point in time.
- Paradoxically, acute, high-intensity exercise appears to improve orthostatic intolerance, while prolonged exercise decreases it. Understanding the interaction with exercise could be modeled theoretically and tested experimentally.

Does the Evidence Report Address Relevant Interactions Among Risks?

To a limited extent, the evidence report considers interactions. The three areas most in need of additional work include thermal, vestibular, and pharmacologic interactions. The risk mitigation plan for orthostatic intolerance is relatively advanced. However, the efficacy of combination therapies is a gap that should be addressed systematically.

This evidence report describes unanticipated drug interactions resulting from combinations of pharmacological interventions that would not routinely be used in terrestrial medicine (for example, akathisia with combined use of midodrine and promethazine). The observation highlights the need to consider countermeasures individually and in the overall context of a treatment plan.

What Is the Overall Readability and Quality?

In general, the evidence report was well organized. The writing is complete. The document is easy to follow and comprehend. However, there are several mislabeled legends and figures. The color codes are reversed for Figure 16.

Is the Breadth of the Cited Literature Sufficient?

For the topics directly covered in this evidence report the cited references were comprehensive. However, it is likely the narrative and supporting references will need to be expanded to adequately address the newly identified knowledge gaps, particularly in the areas of vascular biology and in dynamic monitoring and prediction of impending orthostatic events (e.g., Behnke et al., 2011; Reisner et al., 2011; Stabley et al., 2012; Taylor et al., 2013).

Is the Expertise of the Authors Sufficient to Fully Cover the Scope of the Given Risk? Is Input from Additional Disciplines Needed?

The expertise of the authoring team is appropriate. The cardiovascular descriptions are logical and thorough. Related disciplines that could provide additional insight include pharmacology, vascular biology, statistical validation of modeling techniques, and comparative effectiveness of countermeasures. These interventions need ongoing integration with the skeletal muscle and nutrition evidence base. All of these need to be integrated with the quantification of physiological demands of nominal and emergency tasks.

Has the Evidence Report Addressed Previous Recommendations Made by the IOM in the 2008 Letter Report?

The 2008 report identified the following recommendations:

> A particular concern is the total lack of information about whether partial-gravity exposure (1/6 G on the Moon and 3/8 G on Mars) will exacerbate or mitigate effects against orthostatic intolerance following prolonged spaceflight. Ground-based studies directed toward answering these questions are under way, but it is not clear that these can fully reproduce the effects of prolonged exposure to microgravity in space. To date, an effective countermeasure for orthostatic intolerance has not been fully identified. (p. 54)
>
> The gaps should include preflight fitness requirements for cardiovascular capacity relating to prolonged space travel. Gender

> should also be considered as a potential gap. Although gender-related data are limited, it does point to a potential issue. Gaps … should include cardiac and skeletal muscle mass as potentially important contributors to cardiovascular performance. (p. 55)

Clearly, the evidence base has expanded since the previous review of this area, and the authors should be commended for their regular update of this evidence report. However, as noted above, the fractional gravity area remains a research gap, and the information on exposure durations that inform exploration-class spaceflight risks are also still lacking.

RISK OF INJURY AND COMPROMISED PERFORMANCE DUE TO EVA OPERATIONS

The report *Risk of Injury and Compromised Performance Due to EVA Operations* (Chappell et al., 2015) deals with issues surrounding EVA and is informed by a substantial amount of experience from EVA activities to date. The evidence report provides a strong overview of the relevant issues and describes the complexities of the hazardous environments faced in space exploration and the challenges in designing EVA suits and training regimens to overcome those hazards. This evidence report could be strengthened by additional discussion of alternative suit architectures and other topics outlined in the review that follows.

Does the Evidence Report Provide Sufficient Evidence, as Well as Sufficient Risk Context, That the Risk Is of Concern for Long-Term Space Missions?

The report discusses the issues associated with suit design and presents data from the ISS and Apollo-era experiences; the report also includes results of studies conducted to identify characteristics of future suits to support EVA requirements during expedition-class missions. This evidence report provides a comprehensive review of both the external hazards faced in EVA operations, particularly excessive radiation exposure and unviable breathing environments, as well as the hazards and challenges posed within the microclimate of the space suit such as hypoxia, humidity, suit pressure, and the biological challenges including thermal dysregulation, nutrition and hydration, and waste removal needs. The report, however, lacks specificity concerning the types of EVA tasks that likely will be performed during expeditions to asteroids, the Moon, or Mars.

In addition, the report is predicated on the assumption that gas-pressurized suit architecture (similar to that used during Apollo or on ISS EVAs) is the only option available, and all gaps addressed by the authors derive from this assumption. The rationale for leaving out a consideration of alternative suit architectures, such as the Z-2 gas pressurized suit under development, or a mechanical counter-pressurized (MCP) suit, is not stated.

Does the Evidence Report Make the Case for the Research Gaps Presented?

Seven research gaps are listed in the evidence report (numbered 6 through 11 and 14; Box 2). The committee believes the evidence report authors adequately supported these seven gaps but did not provide justification for retiring previously identified gaps.

BOX 2
Research Gaps Identified in the Evidence Report

- EVA 6: What crew physiological and performance capabilities are required for EVA operations in exploration environments?
- EVA 7: How do EVA suit system design parameters affect crew health and performance in exploration environments?
- EVA 8: What are the physiological inputs and outputs associated with EVA operations in exploration environments?
- EVA 9: What is the effect on crew performance and health of variations in EVA task design and operations concepts for exploration environments?
- EVA 10: Can knowledge and use of real-time physiological and system parameters during EVA operations improve crew health and performance?
- EVA 11: How do EVA operations in exploration environments increase the risk of crew injury and how can the risk be mitigated?
- EVA 14: What other EVA-related risks, developments, and technologies exist that may affect EVA research?

SOURCE: Chappell et al., 2015.

Gaps 1 through 5 and 12 and 13 are not mentioned in the evidence report. The IOM committee found that that gaps 1-5 had been retired by a 2009 Standing Review Panel (NASA, 2015). Gap 13 (EVA 13: What is the risk of hypoxia during exploration missions?) is listed on the NASA website as a current gap but is not included in the evidence report (Chappell et al., 2015; NASA, 2015). Additionally, there may be a re-numbering issue as the website discusses the creation of EVA gaps 6-13 but then lists them as gaps 6-11 and 13-14 (NASA, 2015). The website notes:

> Following the 2009 Standing Review Panel, the EPSP [EVA Physiology, Systems, and Performance] Project conducted an extensive project portfolio review. Subsequently EVA gaps 1-5 were deleted, and EVA gaps 6-13 were created to clarify the areas that should be addressed to mitigate this risk. Applicable tasks from EVA gaps 1-5 (below) were mapped to the new EVA gaps.
>
> - EVA 1: What models and techniques are required to evaluate various suit designs and operational concepts to optimize crew health and performance?
> - EVA 2: What are the physiological and biomechanical stimuli associated with various suit designs and EVA tasks?
> - EVA 3: What suit characteristics, systems, and consumables requirements are needed to optimize crew performance, health and safety?
> - EVA 4: What technologies and in-suit countermeasures can be integrated into the EVA suit to optimize crew performance, health and safety?
> - EVA 5: How can decompression sickness (DCS) risk be characterized, mitigated, and/or treated?

The committee recognizes that the retired gap 5 on decompression sickness has now become a separate risk category with its own evidence report (see discussion beginning on page 31). Further, the Standing Review Panel's revisions focus the new gaps (see Box 2) on the physiological aspects of suit design as related to astronaut health and performance.

However, the committee believes that there is value in noting these changes in the evidence report and retaining the retired gaps by marking them as inactive (or some other similar notation) to ensure that all issues are carefully considered particularly in planning for EVA activities on a planetary surface. Because the evidence reports act as a repository for knowledge about risks and gaps in knowledge, the rationale for changes should be included in the evidence reports. This appears particularly important at a time when future planning for longer duration interplanetary missions will, of necessity, move from a situation of more certainty to one of less certainty.

Are There Any Additional Gaps in Knowledge or Areas of Fundamental Research That Should Be Considered to Enhance the Basic Understanding of This Specific Risk?

Gap 6 in the evidence report asks "What crew physiological and performance capabilities are required for EVA operations in exploration environments?" The report offers metrics to close the gap: aerobic fitness standard; muscle strength and power required; anthropometry; loss of physical function during transit to EVA site; and EVA activity contributing to physiological countermeasures. These are valid issues, but what is missing is a detailed understanding of the work that will be performed by the human crew outside the protection of a space ship or planetary habitat during expedition-class missions. All garments, from running shorts to elaborate protective ensembles are designed with an understanding of the tasks that will be performed while wearing them. The primary research gap missing from many of the NASA evidence reports, including this one, is the need for a systematic analysis of tasks likely to be performed by crew personnel during long-duration space missions. In conjunction with this, a method for evaluation of performance will be needed. Based on information presented in the evidence report, it is possible that the constraints imposed by conventional pressure-suit designs of the type described by the authors, while adequate for ISS EVA activities, might not support the surface operation requirements of planetary expeditions. Only a task analysis will determine the optimal design for suits to be used for EVAs on planetary surfaces. The task analysis will provide insights into the potential concerns and will define the requirements for suits. The optimal design will be defined by evaluating the available technologies and applying human factors design principles.

This evidence report is based on the assumption that gas-pressurized suit architecture is the only option available, and all gaps addressed by the authors derive from this assumption. Much of the gap analysis would be different if EVA gap 1 had not been retired and alternative architectures to conventional gas-pressurized designs had been evaluated in the evidence report. The assumption in the evidence report seems to run counter to NASA's recent expression of interest in MCP garment development; for example, a request for proposals closed in May 2015 for development of flight-ready MCP gloves, indicating an official interest in other approaches. For these reasons, the gaps should be re-evaluated to compare and contrast conventional suit designs with innovative and emerging designs and technologies (including the Z-2 suit and MCP suit). Visionaries, such as Chesley Bonestell (see image, below, illustrating Werner von Braun's plan for Mars exploration), have postulated the need for suits that could accommodate frequent, highly variable EVA requirements (Ley and von Braun, 1956) (see Figure 3).

The major issues missing are the discussions of task-analytic data (a deficit shared by other NASA evidence reports) and discussion of an alternative to conventional EVA suit design. Additional gaps include discussions regarding the mechanisms for mitigating the effects of pressure-suit punctures and the effects of physiological deconditioning on human performance during EVAs in pressure suits. In the absence of task-analytic data, details are not available on the work that will be performed on the surfaces of asteroids and Mars; however, it is reasonable

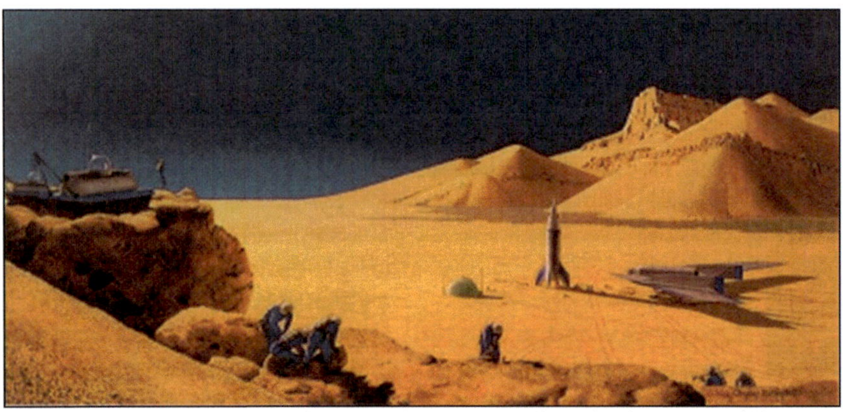

FIGURE 3 An illustration from *Exploring Mars* by Chesley Bonestell, 1956. SOURCE: Reproduced courtesy of Bonestell, LLC.

to assume that geological exploration and construction activities will be involved. In this regard, it is relevant to note that most of the physical injuries sustained by Antarctic analog personnel are trauma to the hands and feet (Stuster, 2010). Many of the injuries sustained in underwater training for EVA are at the shoulder with possible connection to suit design. For this reason, the possibility of abrasion and/or mechanical puncture of suit materials during EVA should be addressed as a research gap as it could have potentially catastrophic consequences for astronaut safety. Similarly, the requirements for considerable muscle strength to operate gas-pressurized suits were established by the evidence report. Potential effects on accomplishing mission objectives, surviving emergencies, and performing contingency operations should be considered.

The evidence report discusses the Apollo EVA experiences in detail, and the committee believes that is appropriate as those 28 EVAs remain the only surface (non-Earth) EVAs to date. The following quotes from a review of the lessons learned during the Apollo missions (Scheuring et al., 2007) highlight some of the limitations of the conventional gas-pressurized suit design.

> According to the Apollo lunar crews, the most fatiguing part of surface EVA tasks was repetitive gripping. Regarding the glove, one crewmember stated, "*Efficiency was no more than 10% of the use of the hand.*" The fingernails generally tended to be pulled back resulting in separation of the nail from the bed, or onycholysis. Additionally, the skin frequently was abraded from the top of the knuckles. This event took on operational and potentially mission significance as several lunar walkers stated that they would not be able to work in the glove beyond the two to three EVAs they completed due to the swelling and pain over the bony prominences of the metacarpal phalangeal (MCP) and proximal interphalangeal (PIP) joints (knuckles), although had they been asked, it is probably that at least one more EVA would have been possible.... Designers should consider a wrist seal and depressurized glove. (p. 8)

> EVA suit mobility was more of an issue in terms of surface locomotion and energy expenditure. The crews often felt they were fighting the resistance in the suit (including in the glove as mentioned above). This was fatiguing, especially in the thighs. The astronauts pointed out that the lunar surface is more similar to an

> ocean than to a desert. The undulating surface posed a number of challenges, including ambulating against a suit that did not allow mobility at the hip. Normal human locomotion includes flexion at the hip and the Apollo A7LB had limited ability to bend the suit at the hip and to rotate within the suit. The crewmember had to bend forward from the knee joint, which demanded considerably more work load on the quadriceps muscles. Therefore, the mobility recommendations centered on adding hip mobility and improved knee flexibility. One comment summed this point well, "*Bending the knee was difficult in the suit. We need a better [more flexible] knee joint.*" Reducing suit pressure to ~3.0 psia (sea-level oxygen partial pressure) with a pure oxygen system would accomplish this to some extent. (p. 9)
>
> EVA suit puncture hazard was a primary concern of the lunar astronauts, although the risk was considered low. Astronauts suggested that protecting suit occupants from a break in suit integrity was appropriate for future research and development activities. However, the trade-offs for this need to be considered carefully relative to mission rules if there is a puncture and emergency regulation of suit pressure and the availability of rover consumables, etc. (p. 10)

Does the Evidence Report Address Relevant Interactions Among Risks?

The evidence report identifies links to the evidence reports on inadequate human–computer interaction, training deficiencies, personnel selection issues, and mostly the risk of decompression sickness. Additional interactions that require attention include

- *Risk of Inadequate Nutrition* (Smith et al., 2015): malnourished astronauts are at risk for physical failure during highly strenuous EVAs,
- *Risk of Reduced Physical Performance Capabilities Due to Reduced Aerobic Capacity* (Downs et al., 2015): EVAs require aerobic stamina due to physicality of tasks, stiffness of gas suit, and

- *Risk of Impaired Performance Due to Reduced Muscle Mass, Strength, and Endurance* (Ploutz-Snyder et al., 2015): EVA requires strength to avoid fatigue and to accomplish EVA objectives.

What Is the Overall Readability and Quality?

The evidence report is well written and understandable even for non-experts, although editing would be helpful. The committee also noted that in several places the differences between underwater training and microgravity were not clearly stated or acknowledged. Underwater (neutral buoyancy) training only partially simulates microgravity because one retains the 1-G gravitational forces on the balance organs and all internal organs. The committee also noted some need to distinguish between weight and inertial mass. Some terms, such as "non-optimized offload kinetics" (p. 8) should be defined.

Is the Breadth of the Cited Literature Sufficient?

Extensive literature is cited, but nothing concerning alternative suit designs is among the references. References that could be added include Webb and Annis, 1967; Webb, 1968; Newman et al., 2005; Waldie, 2005; Holschuh, 2014.

Is the Expertise of the Authors Sufficient to Fully Cover the Scope of the Given Risk? Is Input from Additional Disciplines Needed?

The authors and contributors to the report are all highly qualified experts with expertise in suit design for deep-sea diving, aviation, and spaceflight and with experience in EVAs. Additional input is needed from experts who can evaluate alternative approaches to conventional pressure suits for expedition-class space missions. At the very least, the authors should explain why other approaches to suit design were not mentioned in the report. The issue should be addressed, even if the authors believe that conventional design is the only possible solution to EVA requirements. The effects of radiation on human EVA capability also should be addressed in greater detail, along with actionable strategies for mitigating radiation exposure during EVA.

Has the Evidence Report Addressed Previous Recommendations Made by the IOM in the 2008 Letter Report?

The committee finds it noteworthy that the 2008 letter report made the following recommendations (among others):

1. Reduce the risk of falling through use of better boots, gloves, biosuit (skin-tight suits), auxiliary displays, and navigation and terrain information.
2. Study of alternate joint designs. (p. 51)

The 2008 report also notes, under relevant interactions among risks, "the risk of poor task design. The design of tasks that necessitate EVA must necessarily consider the physical and other limitations created by the suit." The committee notes that the current evidence report reflects and addresses this recommendation, but would also add that the tasks anticipated during planetary surface exploration are in some ways fundamentally different and need careful analysis.

The evidence reports need to clearly distinguish EVAs during planetary surface exploration from in-orbit EVAs. The evidence report authors could consider coining a separate term for EVAs conducted on a planetary surface to distinguish the activity from EVAs conducted in Earth orbit (i.e., freefall or simulated microgravity). A term such as "planetary EVA" or "extra habitat activity" could be used to convey the fundamental differences in environmental conditions and human and equipment requirements.

The committee also highlights the need to ensure that crewmembers be able to be individually distinguished in their spacesuits; color-coding or distinguishing marking will be necessary for asteroid and planetary exploration. During development of the Z-2 suit, another pressurized suit, NASA circulated a large number of photos and drawings, many of which show luminescent patches. These could be color-coded (see Figure 4).

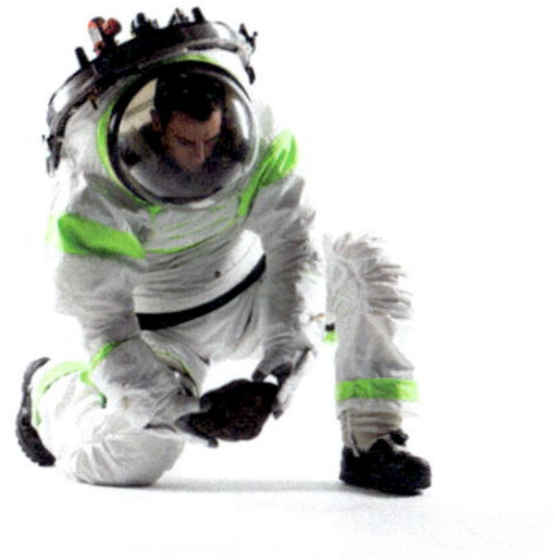

FIGURE 4 Z-2 suit design with luminescent patches.
SOURCE: NASA, 2014b.

RISK OF DECOMPRESSION SICKNESS

Decompression sickness (DCS) is a condition that arises when partial pressures of inert gas in the tissues exceed ambient pressure, resulting in gas bubble formation. These bubbles can cause a variety of medical issues, ranging from localized pain to more severe cardiopulmonary or neurological conditions such as venous and arterial gas emboli, stroke, or even death. During a typical human space mission, the conditions conducive to DCS could occur during an EVA when astronauts are asked to don and then manipulate and ambulate in gas-pressurized space suits that operate at lower ambient pressure levels than the vehicle or habitat. Suit operating pressure is reduced to minimize suit rigidity and maximize mobility—the soft suit materials stiffen when pressurized, making it difficult to articulate the suit joints and causing significant astronaut exertion (and frequently, injury). As a result, suits typically use O_2 gas (rather than air) to maintain sufficient partial pressures of oxygen for respiration in the reduced pressure environment. These conditions—a switch from high- to low-pressure work environment, combined with significant exertion at low pressure during EVA—result in risk for DCS during human space exploration.

The committee reviewed the evidence report *Risk of Decompression Sickness* (Conkin et al., 2013). The report presents a thorough summary of the symptoms, causes, and treatments for DCS, as well as the evidence of (and risk for) DCS during human spaceflight missions.

Does the Evidence Report Provide Sufficient Evidence, as Well as Sufficient Risk Context, That the Risk Is of Concern for Long-Term Space Missions?

Based on our current understanding of the factors contributing to DCS—derived predominantly from experience gained in diving and during high-altitude operations on Earth—the authors provide a clear case for the risk of DCS during future human space exploration EVAs. According to current understanding, as long as astronauts are tasked with conducting EVAs in suits with lower operating pressures than the pressures in their vehicle or habitat, the risk for DCS exists. However, this risk assessment includes two fundamental assumptions:

1. The causal mechanisms for DCS in space are the same as those on Earth (i.e., the understanding of the physiologic response to decompression in micro- or partial-G environments is accurate)
2. EVAs will be conducted in suits at lower operating pressure than the vehicle or habitat.

Based on the evidence provided in the report, it is unclear whether these assumptions are valid. Testing of current astronaut pre-breathe protocols on Earth leads to an expected in-space DCS incidence rate of approximately 20 percent; however, no in-space DCS incidents have been reported in the history of the space program. The source of this discrepancy is not currently understood, although theories are posited in the evidence report (including a lack of symptoms, confusion regarding symptoms, or a lack of willingness to report symptoms).

The assumption that EVAs will be conducted in a low-pressure, gas-pressurized suit, ignores the prospect of alternate suit architectures. For example, MCP suits, such as the Space Activity Suit or the Massachusetts Institute of Technology (MIT) BioSuit, pressurize the wearer using tight fitting materials rather than pressurized gas, enabling suits to operate at higher pressures without necessarily limiting astronaut mobility. As previously noted, NASA is investigating these technologies (e.g., a 2015 call for MCP glove development has been recently awarded), which could have significant implications for future DCS risk in space. This report does not appear to consider such alternatives.

The uncertainty behind these assumptions needs to be resolved in order to know with confidence the magnitude of DCS risk (if any) that needs to be addressed in future human space missions.

Does the Evidence Report Make the Case for the Research Gaps Presented?

The evidence report identifies seven research gaps in DCS knowledge:

DCS 1. We have not defined the acceptable DCS risk with respect to the work efficiency index for exploration scenarios.
DCS 2. We do not know the contribution of specific DCS risk factors to the development of DCS in the spaceflight exploration environment.
DCS 3. We do not know the mission related factors that contribute to DCS risk.
DCS 4. We do not know to what extent physiological and environmental factors can be incorporated and validated in a model of DCS for micro- and reduced gravity.
DCS 5. We do not know what validated procedures will adequately prevent DCS.
DCS 6. We do not know what new developments related to DCS will come from other investigators.
DCS 7. We have not validated procedures to adequately treat DCS in the spaceflight environment should it occur.

These gaps are well supported by the report: fundamental DCS dynamics are poorly understood (e.g., gas bubble formation, growth, and movement), and the existing DCS model and protocols have not been validated for future exploration design reference missions. The committee believes that the gaps listed by NASA outline many (but not all) of the gaps in understanding of the risks associated with DCS in human space exploration. Gap 5 could be restated to be more specific to long-duration/planetary exploration missions, as the current pre-breathe protocols have been used by spacewalkers with no adverse events and a focus is needed on exploring protocols for different environmental conditions, particularly planetary environments. Gap 6 as stated in the evidence report (and listed above) does not point to a specific gap but states an obvious process in science—the potential for new developments. NASA could consider deleting or revising this gap statement.

Are There Any Additional Gaps in Knowledge or Areas of Fundamental Research That Should Be Considered to Enhance the Basic Understanding of This Specific Risk?

The following specific gaps in knowledge are highlighted (in no particular order), some of which may be partially encompassed by the previously enumerated list, and others, which represent new and unique gaps. These gaps warrant additional research to best understand the risk of DCS in human space exploration:

- Task analysis: Specific, mission-focused task analyses are needed for future EVAs in micro- and partial gravity. Future EVAs may more closely resemble Apollo-style surface exploration (characterized by locomotion and full-body activity) than the current paradigm of zero-G, ISS-style EVAs (which consist predominantly of arm/hand manipulations with an anchored lower body). Consequently, it is critical that the set of expected tasks to be performed in future EVAs are established and characterized and that there is an understanding of the energetics of those activities. Knowing that the EVA represents the "altitude" phase of the decompression cycle (when DCS risk is at its highest), expected exertion for EVA tasks needs to be well understood, as it may affect the type and duration of EVA operations that are feasible (or add additional requirements for suit mobility).
- Risk profiles: Information is needed on the composite risk profile for (and variance within) individuals likely to be selected as astronauts on long-duration missions (e.g., middle-aged men and women), so recommendations for crew selection can be based on minimizing risk. It is known that the astronaut population is self-selected to be generally healthy and that the risk of DCS varies in individuals both within and between demographics; however, much remains to be learned about individual variation (e.g., why certain divers are less susceptible to DCS and why some acclimatize, whereas others sensitize in the face of repeat exposure) or what defines an "ideal" demographic for long-duration spaceflight with respect to DCS risk (there may be conflicting "ideal" demographics, depending on which physiological risk is prioritized).
- DCS dynamics: More needs to be understood about the differences, if any, in DCS dynamics in a zero- or partial-G environment compared to a 1-G environment (and the lack of definitive

explanation for the current discrepancy between expected and actual DCS incidents in space). Knowledge of, and protocols for, DCS are necessarily developed and tested in 1-G environments, and to date they have only been operationally validated in microgravity (on the ISS). Experience with planetary EVA is limited, and experience with planetary EVA following a long-duration microgravity transit is nonexistent. Exploring DCS dynamics in varying gravity environments includes examining what, if any, changes these differences have on the risk of DCS onset in these regimes, and what, if any, changes these differences have on Earth-based protocol validation strategies.

- Alternate suit architectures: Cost–benefit analyses are needed of alternate suit architectures with respect to reducing DCS risk. As discussed earlier regarding the EVA evidence report, advanced mobility suit concepts such as MCP suits offer significant advantages over gas-pressurized suits (and can potentially be operated at higher pressures with less effort, decreasing both the difference between vehicle and suit pressure and the energetic cost of EVAs, thereby doubly decreasing DCS risk). While these suits are not operationally viable today, more research needs to be conducted to determine the cost-benefit of advancing MCP technology to flight-level capability.
- Pre-breathe protocols: Specific risks associated with interruptions of otherwise-validated pre-breathe protocols need to be understood. It is clear that these types of interruptions are unavoidable in practice, although little explanation or justification is provided for the established protocol in these cases (two times payback time relative to interruption length, or four times payback time if the break occurs early in the exercise protocol). This area is ripe for additional study enumerating or minimizing likely sources of interruption (i.e., operations); the physiological effects of pre-breathe interruption and the variance in individual response (i.e., physiology); and advanced mitigation strategies with targeted treatments for individuals with differing susceptibility (i.e., advanced technological and medical intervention strategies).
- Technologies: Further understanding how to monitor and diagnose DCS will necessitate reliable, portable, and safe technologies to monitor and diagnose DCS. Previous attempts at in-suit monitoring (venous gas embolism monitoring via in-suit Doppler

detector) were discontinued despite showing promise. The committee recognizes that there are conflicting priorities between incorporation of in-suit technology and reduction of risk of fire within the suit, however the decision to discontinue in-suit monitoring for DCS needs to be revisited because of the potential benefit that such monitoring may offer the astronaut on long-duration missions. Further, the establishment of a reliable biomarker for DCS diagnosis purposes would help immensely in understanding the prevalence of DCS (independent of subjective reporting) and in validation of future pre-breathe protocols.

- Operationally efficient pre-breathe protocols for long-duration missions: Given the complete absence of DCS in space to date, it is theoretically possible that existing protocols could be shortened without compromising safety. The committee encourages NASA to explore this possibility, as a streamlined pre-breathe protocol would enable crew time to be spent on more productive activities.
- DCS treatment: More robust treatment mechanisms should be developed. A detailed strategy for treating moderate-to-severe DCS on a long-duration mission is needed as is the infrastructure necessary to provide treatment should DCS occur. As it stands, the last-ditch response is to over-pressurize the operational EVA suit to provide repressurization, compromising the suit in the process. This is not an acceptable intervention on a deep-space mission, where resupply is impossible, as it puts future EVAs (and therefore mission success) at extreme risk.
- Intra-personal variances throughout long-duration missions: Physiological deconditioning over the course of a long mission may affect an individual's relative DCS susceptibility. Long-duration spaceflight potentially can cause deconditioning and alteration of many physiologic systems (e.g., bone density and muscle mass loss, weakening of cardiac output, fluid shifts, vision changes). Currently it is not known how an individual's specific DCS risk changes as they decondition or how much variance there is in individual risk for a given change in these physiologic systems. These interrelated effects, which may manifest part way through a long-duration mission, warrant additional study to understand their effect on total DCS risk.

Does the Evidence Report Address Relevant Interactions Among Risks?

The report is thorough, and through the discussion provided by the authors, interactions are frequently addressed. Table 6 (Individual Factors Associated with Risk of DCS and Venous Gas Emboli, p. 39) of the report enumerates several known risk factors for DCS (age, patent foramen ovale [a relatively common and generally benign defect of the heart involving a passage in the heart wall], sex, menstrual cycle time, aerobic fitness, body fat, hydration systems). The committee concurs with these risk factors, and volunteers additional relevant interactions based on other evidence reports compiled by NASA, including

- *Risk of Injury and Compromised Performance Due to EVA Operations* (Chappell et al., 2015)
- *Risk of Inadequate Task Design* (Sándor et al., 2013)
- *Risk of Reduced Physical Performance Capabilities Due to Reduced Aerobic Capacity* (Downs et al., 2015)
- *Risk of Impaired Performance Due to Reduced Muscle Mass, Strength, and Endurance* (Ploutz-Snyder et al., 2015)
- *Risk of Performance Decrement and Crew Illness Due to Inadequate Food System* (Perchonok et al., 2012)
- *Risk of Inadequate Nutrition* (Smith et al., 2015)
- *Risk of Unacceptable Health and Mission Outcomes Due to Limitations of In-Flight Medical Capabilities* (Archibald and Kelleher, 2015)

In the committee's opinion, these are relevant risk interactions because they include those with a direct effect on DCS risk (e.g., suit systems and EVA task allocation), those which systemically decondition the astronaut which may increase his or her susceptibility to DCS (e.g., environmentally induced issues such as cardiac and muscle loss, as well as nutrition-induced issues), and those with a direct effect on DCS treatment (e.g., lack of in-flight treatment capabilities).

What Is the Overall Readability and Quality?

The report is of high quality—it is scholarly, complete, well written, and the conclusions follow from the data presented. Two small points of confusion in equations presented in the evidence report were identified.

First, Equation 1 (p. 7) needs to be clarified (Conkin et al., 2013). The committee has previously seen the supersaturation equation formulated differently (Davis et al., 2008, p. 56):

$$\text{Supersaturation} = \sum P_g + \sum P_v - \sum P_a$$

where P_g is the sum of the tensions of all dissolved gases; P_v is the sum of vapor pressures; and P_a is local absolute pressure. This appears to be a slightly different statement than Equation 1 in the evidence report. Are they equivalent, or should Equation 1 in the report be updated?

Second, the bubble growth equation (defined on page 22 of the evidence report) contains the following term. This term has also been written without the negative sign in previous evidence reports (Gernhardt et al., 2009, p. 351).

$$\frac{-\alpha D}{h(r,t)}$$

This confusion highlights the necessity to carefully reference key material such as equations used to model complex systems.

Is the Breadth of the Cited Literature Sufficient?

The report carries an impressive bibliography, with more than 230 sources cited. However, the committee concurs with the 2014 DCS Risk Standing Review Panel (Steinberg et al., 2014) that additional literature review areas could strengthen the report:

- Work by Thom and colleagues at University of Maryland on micronuclei particles
- Work by Flagg and colleagues on pre-breathe interruption
- Work by the U.S. Navy at the Navy Experimental Diving Unit and Naval Submarine Research Lab relating to EVA operations and limited resource allocation
- Reports on the U.S. Air Force Manned Orbital Laboratory Program focusing on manned long-term low-pressure exposures
- Specific research related to U2-pilot DCS (e.g., Pilmanis et al., 2010; Jersey et al., 2013; McGuire et al., 2013)

- A review of research focusing on human adaptation to hypoxic and high-altitude environments
- Work on pre-breathe interruption (Pilmanis et al., 2010; Conkin, 2011)
- Work by Buckey and colleagues on DCS instrumentation (Buckey et al., 2005)

Please refer to the 2014 DCS Standing Review Panel for detailed citation suggestions (Mahon et al., 2014).

Is the Expertise of the Authors Sufficient to Fully Cover the Scope of the Given Risk? Is Input from Additional Disciplines Needed?

The committee believes that the expertise of the authoring team is more than sufficient to cover this topic area. The team has a deep and diversified range of backgrounds and expertise (including physicians, DCS researchers, and EVA and suit experts). The authoring team for the evidence report has done a good job interfacing with additional disciplines to assess DCS risk. As described earlier, due to the significant effect of both space suit architecture and EVA task selection on DCS risk, the committee encourages the DCS community and EVA suit and operations communities to continue working closely to mitigate this risk. Further, because of the difficulty and uncertainty in assessing and treating DCS in situ, the authors are encouraged to more closely interact with the medical and space technology communities on sensing (e.g., in-suit wearable technologies such as venous gas emboli Doppler sensors, or reliable biomarkers) and treatment protocols and technologies (e.g., repressurization suits or Gamow bags).

Has the Evidence Report Addressed Previous Recommendations Made by the IOM in the 2008 Letter Report?

DCS was not included as an independent risk in the 2008 IOM report, but it was included in Chapter 8 "Compromised EVA Performance and Crew Health Due to Inadequate EVA Suit Systems." The committee feels that in pulling DCS out as a separate risk, NASA has responded to the spirit of the 2008 report.

RISK OF PERFORMANCE DECREMENT AND CREW ILLNESS DUE TO AN INADEQUATE FOOD SYSTEM

The risks in the NASA evidence report *Risk of Performance Decrement and Crew Illness Due to an Inadequate Food System* (Perchonok et al., 2012) are broken down into three components: inadequate food safety, inadequate nutritional content of food and intake, and inadequate acceptability of food. Evidence of constraining food system resources was also presented.

Does the Evidence Report Provide Sufficient Evidence, as Well as Sufficient Risk Context, That the Risk Is of Concern for Long-Term Space Missions?

As mission length increases and return to Earth becomes impossible at specific points, the closed system nature of the food supply becomes an increasingly pressing concern. While the feasibility of growing plants in space has been demonstrated on the ISS, it appears likely that any long-duration mission beyond low Earth orbit must pack sufficient food for the journey. The evidence report demonstrates sufficient evidence that this risk is of concern.

Food Safety

Food safety is of concern on Earth and in space. However, the risk associated with food safety issues can potentially be more catastrophic in space. Without information on intervention or cure protocols and the training that astronauts receive, the true severity of the risk cannot be assessed. Additionally, the risk could be higher in space if package integrity may be compromised to a greater extent during spaceflight than on Earth due to physical, thermal, or radiation exposures. The risk could also be higher if thermophilic spoilage microorganisms could grow during transportation or storage which would not normally occur on Earth. The risk associated with the presence of food waste and use of alternative technologies (for producing some foods on the mission) such as hydroponics can increase safety concerns, and these are addressed in the evidence report.

Nutritional Content of Food and Intake

Weight loss for astronauts has been documented in a number of previous space missions (Perchonok et al., 2012). Inadequacy of nutrients provided in Apollo missions in comparison to required levels of nutrients has been documented as discussed in the evidence report, as have decreased levels of vitamins and minerals in blood, urine, and serum. Significant changes in nutrient levels during extended storage has also been documented, and studies of nutrient losses during controlled storage are ongoing.

Acceptability

The level of consumption of food is related to the acceptability of the food. Debriefing of crewmembers has indicated the need for variety in types of food to enhance mood and consumption of the food. Additionally, foods were pre-positioned at the ISS and a decrease in the number of crewmembers sent to the ISS resulted in 3-year-old foods remaining on site and needing to be consumed, thereby causing a decrease in acceptability and consumption of the food. Long-term use effects for defined diets still need to be assessed.

Constraining Food System Resources

People are used to consuming certain foods when they are hot and certain foods when they are cold. However, systems for heating and cooling foods may not be readily available during spaceflight due to weight and volume constraints. The need for heating and cooling of foods to make them acceptable has been documented based on interviews with crew.

One common factor that has not been adequately addressed in this evidence report is the relationship between any of the factors discussed and the level of performance of required tasks. A concerted coordinated effort is needed.

Does the Evidence Report Make the Case for the Research Gaps Presented?

The evidence report details the following research gaps and provides the evidence and the concerns regarding each of these gaps:

- *AFT1: How can the food system deliver the required level of nutrition throughout the mission?*
- *AFT2: How can the nutrition and acceptability of the food system be maintained throughout the mission?*
- *AFT3: How can the acceptability of the food system be maintained throughout the mission?*
- *AFT4: What technologies can be developed that will efficiently balance appropriate vehicle resources such as mass, volume, and crewtime during exploration missions with the safety, nutrition, and acceptability requirements?* (Perchonok et al., 2012, p. 5)

The report discusses the issues regarding kinetic models available to date that are not accurate enough to predict the true shelf life of a given product, especially under extended storage time at the intended conditions for long-duration missions. Additionally, the models indicate that several of the existing foods deemed acceptable for current space missions will not be acceptable for longer duration missions. This justifies the need for exploring alternative technologies for preparing, processing, packaging, and storing foods and also developing more accurate models for predicting the shelf life of products. Such models can make use of the 2 to 3 additional years of the storage study data collected by NASA (Cooper et al., 2011) as well as the ongoing storage study of similar military ration items that are under way at the U.S. Army Laboratories in Natick, Massachusetts. Ongoing communications and collaborations with the Natick research team are encouraged.

The need to develop methods to minimize the residual level of oxygen within a package has been properly identified in the evidence report. The need for developing high-barrier packaging materials that are lightweight and easily disposed has also been appropriately addressed.

Food waste and packaging waste have been documented in the evidence report to be a leading category of waste during space exploration missions. Thus, the need to develop strategies to minimize these is evident. The need to develop bioregenerative systems has been mentioned.

This section could be strengthened with appropriate references on the technologies that are currently available.

The possibility of using probiotics to potentially enhance the health and well-being of crewmembers was mentioned. However, data on survival of these probiotics during extended periods of time are needed as are data on the link between probiotics and preventing illness (and improving performance).

Are There Any Additional Gaps in Knowledge or Areas of Fundamental Research That Should Be Considered to Enhance the Basic Understanding of This Specific Risk?

Understanding Food Safety and Processing Technologies

Although inadequate food safety was listed as a concern, it has not been listed as one of the areas of fundamental research that should be conducted in the list of gaps at the bottom of page 5 of the evidence report. Perhaps there was a typo or some duplication between gaps 2 and 3 (p. 5). Safety assurance measures currently in place for prepackaged foods on spaceflights were well covered. However, growing or processing foods from bulk ingredients during the mission do present challenges. For example, some dry ingredients previously thought to be safe have been found to harbor surviving *Salmonella* species that can cause illness (Finn et al., 2013). Added safety assurance measures or improved processes should be investigated for some basic ingredients such as milk, egg powders, or flour.

The shelf life and quality of a product depend on the ingredients used, processing technologies adopted, packaging employed, and storage conditions (EUFIC, 2013). Developing and using high-quality ingredients could potentially result in the production of nutrient dense foods with acceptable nutritional value and shelf life. However, it is also important to understand how bioavailability and bioaccessibility of these nutrients are affected by storage in space or a planetary surface. A reexamination of freeze-dried foods, especially for items to be used in congregate meals, should be conducted with a look at ingredients that may minimize cross-linking that inhibits rehydration during extended storage. Such items can achieve a 5-year shelf life when packaged in high-barrier packaging (Perchonok et al., 2003). The use of emerging rapid heating processes (with ohmic, microwave, or radio frequency technologies), short holding, and rapid cooling or other alternative sterilization technologies, including irradiation (Josephson, 2015), which has been used on previous space missions, could result in improved product quality with longer shelf life. The development of lightweight high-barrier edible films can address shelf life and waste issues simultaneously (Cooper et al., 2011). Additionally, it is important to understand the mechanisms behind the loss in integrity of a package due to physical, thermal, and radiation effects during transportation and storage. Understanding the effect of storing a product at extremely low temperatures that could be found in parts of the space vehicle is important in determining if this option could yield the desired quality and shelf life for a product for long-duration missions.

Fundamental studies addressing the understanding of the kinetics of detrimental reactions, including oxidation and cross-linking of food macromolecules during long-term storage and developing the appropriate accelerated shelf life studies should be conducted. The use of time–temperature integrators to monitor product quality and acceptability during missions could help bridge the gap between existing kinetic models and reality. Effect of factors other than temperature (such as radiation exposure during flight or on planetary surfaces) on shelf life should also be considered.

One of the issues that was mentioned in the report is the potential for partial gravity to affect heat and mass transfer for preparation or processing of foods. Conducting mathematical modeling studies would be one way to address this issue to assess if the changes pose safety or quality issues.

Another gap in information relates to appetite and satiety. A thorough investigation on what causes loss of appetite in space is warranted, which should include the effects of taste and flavor perception in space. The types of foods that are preferred during spaceflights may be quite different from those on Earth. The use of nanotechnology to increase the surface area or encapsulation of desirable sensory markers (such as spices or flavors) could enhance the acceptability of foods (Sekhon, 2010).

The use of three dimensional printing can enhance the variety and freshness of foods that might be produced during long-term missions. It is important to understand how this approach could affect food safety, morale, time of preparation of food, and overall acceptability.

Impact on Human Performance

One of the hypotheses in the report relates to performance decrement of crew as a result of lower levels of nutrition and calories. To substantiate this hypothesis, it would be appropriate to develop the benchmarks for the nutritional and caloric needs to perform various tasks and also quantify how performance decreases as nutritional and caloric intakes decrease below the threshold values. Here, the Food Systems group could profitably work with the NASA Nutrition Research group and consult the published research on nutrition and human performance conducted by U.S. Army researchers. One such reference (Friedl and Hoyt, 1997) is cited in the evidence report.

Utilization of Waste

Research on the use of waste generated in space, especially on planetary surfaces, should be conducted. This includes both food waste and packaging waste. Solid waste could potentially be used to generate energy, liquid waste could be reclaimed as potable water, and packaging waste could potentially be used to shield against radiation or other uses. Consideration should be given to exploring improved packaging of foods for long-duration missions that would have inner nonstick coatings to minimize adherence of food to the package, thereby maximizing food consumption and minimizing waste and the safety concerns associated with residual food.

Research on developing lighter heating and cooling devices should be investigated so as to increase the acceptability of foods by maintaining foods hot or cold, as desired. This could involve research on Peltier-effect systems or thermoelectric generators.

Does the Evidence Report Address Relevant Interactions Among Risks?

Interaction effects between microgravity, radiation, temperature, and time on the safety, quality, and acceptability of foods has been hypothesized. However, the quantification of the effects has not been done. Additionally, the interaction between payload constraints on the ability to prepare, store, or serve foods and the acceptability of foods (both from a nutritional and a sensory standpoint) has not been appropriately addressed.

The availability of sufficient potable water for drinking and food preparation at each stage of the missions should not be overlooked.

What Is the Overall Readability and Quality?

Overall the report is well written and the information is clearly and logically presented. However, information on newer processing and preparation technologies is somewhat lacking in the report because of the time lag from the report's preparation in 2012 to current date. This is an area of rapidly evolving technologies and all efforts to update the evidence report as often as possible would be useful.

Is the Breadth of the Cited Literature Sufficient?

Based on the date of the report, the breadth of the cited literature is appropriate. However, since the report was prepared more than 2 years ago, there have been several key developments, especially in the area of food-processing technologies. The most recent citations from 2012 were all internal NASA reports. Additional details on these focal areas have been given in the question above that addresses additional gaps.

Is the Expertise of the Authors Sufficient to Fully Cover the Scope of the Given Risk? Is Input from Additional Disciplines Needed?

Together the authors have a combination of technical, experiential, and historical knowledge to adequately address the issue under consideration.

Input from engineering and chemistry (from the standpoint of understanding kinetics of deteriorative reactions, the rate of heat transfer, and extent of mass transfer during transportation and storage) and behavioral sciences (from the standpoint of understanding the relationship between types of foods, change in preferences during spaceflight and microgravity, and the effect of a different social environment on satiety and well-being) could be beneficial in formulating the appropriate types of foods. Understanding the link between level and timing of exercise and sleep on quantity of food intake (and hence, nutritional intake) could be beneficial. Further, communications between the Food Systems and Nutrition Research evidence report teams could improve the joint focus on food and nutrient intake on human performance and behavior.

Has the Evidence Report Addressed Previous Recommendations Made by the IOM in the 2008 Letter Report?

This risk did not appear as a separate chapter to be addressed by the 2008 letter report. The closest identifiable risk, "Chapter 12 Inadequate Nutrition," maps to the corresponding report (see below). The committee feels that creating a separate risk and associated evidence report is an appropriate response to the spirit of the 2008 report.

RISK FACTOR OF INADEQUATE NUTRITION

The need for adequate nutrition, particularly for long-term space missions, is self-evident and complex. What is challenging in addressing this topic is how to cover the breadth and depth of the many areas of nutrition while focusing in on the most relevant issues regarding the risks for long duration space missions.

Does the Evidence Report Provide Sufficient Evidence, as Well as Sufficient Risk Context, That the Risk Is of Concern for Long-Term Space Missions?

The focus of answering this question shifts to whether the evidence report (Smith et al., 2015) provides sufficient risk context and specific relevance to spaceflight, particularly for long-term missions where most foods will be packaged shelf-stable items. Due to the breadth of the topics this report has to address, it is important to strengthen the report's focus on the impact of nutrition on human performance during long-term missions and to clarify throughout the report whether the experimentally derived nutrient data discussed is referencing in vitro, animal, or human data.

Does the Evidence Report Make the Case for the Research Gaps Presented?

Data are provided to make the case for research gaps presented in the evidence report, however in some cases the evidence is overstated (for example, the statement "Abundant data show that eicosapentaenoic acid can successfully prevent muscle atrophy in other muscle-wasting circumstances, such as cancer or sepsis (134-140, 143)" [Smith et al., 2015, p.

31]). This assertion is supported by eight citations; all include the same author and one is a study in children. The relevance of these references to different stresses encountered in long-term space missions needs to be examined. The section on essential fatty acids, especially the omega-3 fatty acids with their wide physiological impact, needs to be updated (see, for example, Jonas and Montain, 2014).

The evidence report is uneven in its descriptions of nutrients and their risks of deficiencies or excesses. For example, folate deficiency is said to be "catastrophic" but not deficiencies of other equally essential nutrients. Risks for nutrient deficiencies seem overstated with worst case of death predominating. The real risk would seem to be in performance decrements from inadequate intake of nutrients.

Dated and incorrect assertions need to be updated. For example, the report asserts "toxic levels of fat lead to high serum cholesterol, obesity, atherosclerotic plaques, and, ultimately, coronary heart disease, or even death" (p. 32). However, fat has not been found to be toxic, and nutritionists generally do not recommend low-fat diets anymore (McManus et al., 2001; USDA/HHS, 2015). Moreover, total fat intake is only weakly associated with obesity. Overall deficient caloric intake or water intakes seem to be dominant risks. One suggestion would be to focus on those nutrients with intakes on space missions of some duration shown in the tables in the evidence report's appendix that are either above (sodium, phosphorous) or below (vitamin D, vitamin E, total calories) standards for space flight.

As presented, the evidence report does not appear to have any consistent criteria for citations, as primary studies are mixed in with reviews and commentaries, and narrative reviews with systematic reviews. Much of the data cited in the report have been derived from short-term spaceflights or bed rest without an explicit attempt to address the issues that would be associated with long-term flights, and some assertions related to short-term effects have since been debunked by longer-term studies. Statistical significance is frequently noted in the report, but assessment of whether such statistically significant differences have biological importance is largely absent. Some of the shortcomings of bed rest studies are mentioned, but weighting of their evidence is not critically addressed.

The report frames the importance of inadequate nutrition in a microgravity environment but does not mention other stressful aspects of spaceflight that will affect human metabolism and the need for optimal nutritional support (e.g., radiation, isolation, or confinement) that have relevance to nutritional requirements. These can be important because they may affect reactive oxygen species, also mentioned in the report. In addition, interaction of the stresses may create effects that are different than any of the stresses alone, and this is not discussed.

Research gaps are presented without any attempt to prioritize their importance. The report would be strengthened by stripping out data that are not corroborated by long-term studies. Indeed almost all the 24 micronutrients discussed have the identical gaps identified, that their content and stability in space foods are unknown. The evidence report on Food Systems discussed above (Perchonok et al., 2012) notes that progress is being made in conducting nutritional analyses. The Nutrition evidence report would greatly benefit from including more evidence on nutrient stability in food and supplements from the NASA food systems team and relevant data on storage stability of nutrients in combat rations from studies being done at the U.S. Army laboratories in Natick, Massachusetts.

The negativity evident in the report with respect to supplements other than vitamin D may not be appropriate, particularly for long-duration missions where fresh fruits and vegetables will not be available. This should be re-examined, especially in regard to water-soluble labile nutrients for which excess doses are not physiologically harmful.

The field of nutrition is moving rapidly, and the report as written is a traditional and somewhat dated catalog of properties of nutrients. It would benefit by updating to include the current state of knowledge about the following:

- Nutrient stability in food, together with evidence of absorption, bioavailability, and bioactivity
- Nutrients (e.g., omega-3 fatty acids and certain amino acids or their metabolites) operating as signaling molecules to influence metabolic pathways and the transcriptional regulation of the genome
- C-1 metabolism and its role in metabolism and gene regulation
- Cofactors of methylation, vitamin B12 and folate, and the ignored methyl donors especially choline (declared an essential nutrient by the IOM in 1998) and the amino acid methionine, and other sulfur compounds (Zeisel et al., 2003; IOM, 2006; Zeisel and da Costa, 2009; Zeisel and Caudill, 2010; Zeisel and Corbin, 2012)
- Effects of omega-3 fatty acids as well as the dietary omega-3 to omega-6 ratio on diverse stress and inflammatory responses and

interaction with high protein diets on renal stone formation (Jonas and Montain, 2014)

- Inclusion of the lessons learned in clinical experience with total parenteral nutrition and in military nutrition research starting with the pioneering nutrition research of C. Frank Consolazio and colleagues in the 1940s carried into the present day. Many major thrusts are captured in published reports of the IOM Committee on Military Nutrition Research (IOM, 1999)
- Effects resulting from studies of timing of food intake relative to exercise, and nutritional effects of circadian shifts and sleep habits

Are There Any Additional Gaps in Knowledge or Areas of Fundamental Research That Should Be Considered to Enhance the Basic Understanding of This Specific Risk?

Behavioral health is not adequately covered in the report, and additional understanding is needed of the inflight biochemical and psychosocial factors that contribute to appetite, palatability and taste perception, satiety, and astronauts not consuming available foodstuffs completely. These factors will be especially important in deciding feeding strategies for long missions that may include planetary exploration missions. A relevant study not referenced was conducted by the IOM Committee on Military Nutrition Research, *Not Eating Enough, Overcoming Underconsumption of Military Operational Rations* (IOM, 1995).

Additional gaps that should be considered include the following:

- Nutritional effects of altered microbiota, particularly for nutrients such as vitamin K that are acquired primarily from microbial metabolism rather than from diet.
- The overall health effects of interactions among nutrients, diet patterns, astronaut nutrition preflight baselines, and personal choices regarding diet. For example, Mediterranean and Western diets of similar nutrient composition have divergent long-term effects on cardiovascular health.
- Individual variation in binding affinities for some needed enzymes (e.g., thiamine and thiamine phosphate coenzyme) as well as the metabolism and absorption of certain micronutrients (e.g., vitamin B12 and choline).

Does the Evidence Report Address Relevant Interactions Among Risks?

Risk interactions are described, but they would be strengthened by addressing the following additional interactions. Food consumed by astronauts in inflight environments may result in altered microbiota, which in turn can have physiologically important effects. These include the possibility of inflammation of specific sites (such as the intestines), which would potentially affect muscle loss, bone loss, and other physiological systems. The microbiome also has known effects on the immune system, and emerging data suggests that there may be effects on neural impulses and resulting influence on brain function. Thus, the addition of interactions with the risks of altered immune function and altered microbial physiology and virulence would be useful. Further, the potential for interactions with the risks noted in other evidence reports could be added, including

- *Risk of Impaired Performance Due to Reduced Muscle Mass, Strength, and Endurance* (Ploutz-Snyder et al., 2015),
- *Risk of Injury and Compromised Performance Due to EVA Operations* (Chappell et al., 2015),
- *Risk of Performance Decrement and Crew Illness Due to an Inadequate Food System* (Perchonok et al., 2012), and
- *Risk of Performance and Behavioral Health Decrements Due to Inadequate Cooperation, Coordination, Communication, and Psychosocial Adaptation Within a Team* (Landon et al., 2015).

What Is the Overall Readability and Quality?

The report as written has the character of two separate catalogs (one written from the perspective of individual nutrients, one from a body systems perspective) simply being concatenated, with substantial duplication across the sections, and lacking narrative that puts into perspective the actual (versus theoretical) inflight risks associated with inadequate nutrition. While a large list or catalog is useful for knowledgeable researchers as a reference resource, the report in its current form lacks perspective and does not serve one of the uses of the evidence reports, which is to engage new generations of researchers and students in solving the health challenges associated with spaceflight. The purpose would be served more effectively by a much shorter version of the first section focused on key issues of dietary content, intake, and stability where risks of nutritional deficits on human performance are highest. As noted above, there is no synthesis of nutrient level data with equally important issues of nutrient interactions and diet. In this regard, food groups could be broken down into groups of nutrient sources to determine whether astronauts can be assured of getting sufficient amounts in long-duration missions.

Statistically significant differences are commonly included in data cited in the report, without addressing whether such differences are biologically significant.

Is the Breadth of the Cited Literature Sufficient?

The report contains 1,032 references, which in some areas is excessive. Given the breadth of the literature, the reference list could be revised to include only key references. There were references dated as late as 2014 in the later sections of the report that dealt with nutrient effects on different aspects of physiology, but stress physiology including oxidative stress and antioxidant impacts were someone dated and missing key elements. For example, glutathione along with vitamin C, vitamin E, and selenium are the most physiologically relevant antioxidants but no consideration of glutathione and nutrient precursors was given.

Is the Expertise of the Authors Sufficient to Fully Cover the Scope of the Given Risk? Is Input from Additional Disciplines Needed?

In a narrow sense, that of classes of nutrients and standard dietary requirements, author expertise is clearly sufficient. A more holistic view of nutrition and the factors that influence it, particularly for long-duration missions, will profit from including expertise in behavioral science and contemporary molecular biology that affects human metabolism, especially in the area of responses to diverse stresses.

Understanding of the relationship between individual nutrient intake and overall individual diet patterns would benefit from contributions by behavioral health researchers. Additional input from physiologists and biochemists studying the effects of phytochemicals on human metabolism, especially in the inflammatory response, is needed to design diets for long-term spaceflight that will confer the benefits that adequate intake of fruits and vegetables provide. Certain supplements using extracts of fruits and vegetables in stable forms that could be made into beverages or other consumable forms should be considered.

Has the Evidence Report Addressed Previous Recommendations Made by the IOM in the 2008 Letter Report?

The 2008 report noted the following challenges with this evidence report that have not been addressed to date.

> Although the document covers evidence regarding 31 nutrients, it does not explain how this list was generated. Therefore it is difficult to know whether these 31 factors were selected from a larger list or if these are all the possible nutrients that could be considered. From the lay perspective, the list would be exhaustive and possibly unnecessary due to the varying levels of strength in the arguments for each. This could be partially clarified by including a review of the current nutritional guidelines used for astronauts and relevant gaps in knowledge associated with each standard. (IOM, 2008, p. 59)
>
> An enormous amount of evidence is reviewed regarding nutrition and previous spaceflights, and it seems likely that that information could be condensed and summarized. (IOM, 2008, p. 60)

SUMMARY

This is the third of five letter reports that will review the entire series of NASA's evidence reports on human health risks. This letter report reviewed seven evidence reports and provided the committee's responses to the questions detailed in the statement of task. The evidence reports are quite thorough in their review of the evidence of spaceflight risks, although they vary in format and in the consistency and quality of the writing. In general, the reports would benefit from the perspectives of authors from more diverse fields and from adding authors from outside of NASA staff and contractors.

Many of these reports cover broad fields of research, and the committee appreciates the challenges in identifying and summarizing the most salient literature. Challenges also arise in finding the best way to highlight the interactions between risks. The reports do an adequate job of discussing the interactions between those risks that are most directly related, but they struggle with establishing the connections and interactions among risks that are related, but a bit more tangential (e.g., relation of nutrition and food supply to many of the other risks such as muscle performance).

In most of the evidence reports that were reviewed, it was evident that the tasks to be accomplished during exploration class missions need to be better defined and need to be incorporated in the evidence reports so that the nature and extent of the risks can be fully explored. The distinctions between EVAs performed on board the ISS and the EVAs that would be performed on planetary surfaces appear to be so significant that the committee suggests different terminology be employed. In the EVA and DCS reports, the committee notes that only one kind of suit architecture is considered. The committee recommends that the risks be more fully explored and the possibility of other types of suit architecture be considered. Finally, individual variability (both positive and negative) is not adequately addressed (e.g., in the reports on DCS and orthostasis).

The committee greatly appreciates the opportunity to review the evidence reports and applauds NASA's commitment to improving the quality of its reports. The evidence reports provide the basis for the work of NASA's Human Research Program, and the in-depth review that they provide will contribute to improving the health and performance of future astronauts and enhancing future human spaceflights endeavors.

Sincerely,

Carol E. H. Scott-Conner, *Chair*
Daniel R. Masys, *Vice Chair*
Committee to Review NASA's Evidence Reports
on Human Health Risks

REFERENCES

Archibald, R., and K. Kelleher. 2015. *NASA evidence report: Risk of unacceptable health and mission outcomes due to limitations of in-flight medical capabilities.* https://humanresearchwiki.jsc.nasa.gov/index.php?title=Exploration_Medical_Capability_(ExM)_Evidence_Report (accessed October 2, 2015).

Behnke, B. J., R. B. Armstrong, and M. D. Delp. 2011. Adrenergic control of vascular resistance varies in muscles composed of different fiber types: Influence of the vascular endothelium. *American Journal of Physiology: Regulatory, Integrative, and Comparative Physiology* 301(3):R783-R790.

Buckey, Jr., H. C., D. A. Knaus, D. L. Alvarenga, M. A. Kenton, and P. J. Magari. 2005. Dual-frequency ultrasound for detecting and sizing bubbles. *Acta Astronautica* 56(9-12):1041-1047.

Chappell, S. P., J. R. Norcross, A. F. J. Abercromby, and M. L. Gernhardt. 2015. *NASA evidence report: Risk of injury and compromised performance due to EVA operations.* http://humanresearchroadmap.nasa.gov/evidence/reports/EVA.pdf (accessed September 29, 2015).

Conkin, J. 2011. Decompression sickness after air break in prebreathe described with a survival model. *Aviation, Space, and Environmental Medicine* 82(6):589-598.

Conkin, J., J. R. Norcross, J. H. Wessel III, A. F. J. Abercromby, J. S. Klein, J. P. Dervay, and M. L. Gernhardt. 2013. *NASA evidence report: Risk of decompression sickness.* http://humanresearchroadmap.nasa.gov/evidence/reports/DCS.pdf (accessed September 29, 2015).

Convertino, V. A., S. A. Bloomfield, and J. E. Greenleaf. 2010. An overview of the issues: Physiological effects of bed rest and restricted physical activity. *Medicine and Science in Sports and Exercise* 29(2):187-190.

Cooper, M., G. Douglas, and M. Perchonok. 2011. Developing the NASA food system for long-duration missions. *Journal of Food Science* 76(2):R40-R48.

Davis, J. R., R. Johnson, J. Stepanek, and J. A. Fogardty, eds. 2008. *Fundamentals of aerospace medicine*, 4th ed. Philadelphia, PA: Lippincott Williams and Wilkins.

Downs, M., A. Moore, S. M. C. Lee, and L. Ploutz-Snyder. 2015. *NASA evidence report: Risk of reduced physical performance capabilities due to reduced aerobic capacity.* http://humanresearchroadmap.nasa.gov/evidence/reports/Aerobic.pdf (accessed September 29, 2015).

EUFIC (European Union Food Information Council). 2013. *Food shelf life and its importance for consumers.* http://www.eufic.org/article/en/artid/Food_shelf_life_and_its_importance_for_consumers (accessed November 11, 2015).

Finn, S., O. Condell, P. McClure, A. Amézquita, and S. Fanning. 2013. Mechanisms of survival, responses and sources of *Salmonella* in low-moisture environments. *Frontiers in Microbiology* 4:331.

Friedl, K. E., and R. W. Hoyt. 1997. Development and biomedical testing of military operational rations. *Annual Review of Nutrition* 17:51-75.

Gernhardt, M. L., J. A. Jones, R. A. Scheuring, A. F. Abercromby, J. A. Tuxhorn, and J. R. Norcross. 2009. Risk of compromised EVA performance and crew health due to inadequate EVA suit systems. In *Human health and performance risks of space exploration missions: Evidence reviewed by the NASA Human Research Program*, edited by J. C. McPhee and J. B. Charles. Washington, DC: Government Printing Office. Pp. 333-358.

Guinet, P., S. M. Schneider, B. R. Macias, D. E. Watenpaugh, R. L. Hughson, A. P. Le Traon, J. Y. Bansard, and A. R. Hargens. 2009. WISE-2005: Effect of aerobic and resistive exercises on orthostatic tolerance during 60 days bed rest in women. *European Journal of Applied Physiology* 106(2):217-227.

Hickson, R. C., C. Kanakis, Jr., J. R. Davis, A. M. Moore, and S. Rich. 1982. Reduced training duration effects on aerobic power, endurance, and cardiac growth. *Journal of Applied Physiology: Respiratory, Environmental and Exercise Physiology* 53(1):225-229.

Hickson, R. C., S. M. Overland, and K. A. Dougherty. 1984. Reduced training frequency on aerobic power and muscle adaptations in rats. *Journal of Applied Physiology: Respiratory, Environmental and Exercise Physiology* 57(6):1834-1841.

Hickson, R. C., C. Foster, M. L. Pollock, T. M. Galassi, and S. Rich. 1985. Reduced training intensities and loss of aerobic power, endurance, and cardiac growth. *Journal of Applied Physiology* 58(2):492-499.

Holschuh, B. T. 2014. *Mechanical counter-pressure space suit design using active materials.* Cambridge, MA: Massachusetts Institute of Technology. http://dspace.mit.edu/handle/1721.1/90602 (accessed October 2, 2015).

Huguet, A., J. A. Hayden, J. Stinson, P. J. McGrath, C. T. Chambers, M. E. Tougas, and L. Wozney. 2013. Judging the quality of evidence in reviews of prognostic factor research: Adapting the GRADE framework. *Systematic Reviews* 2(1):71.

Hunter, S. K. 2014. Sex differences in human fatigability: Mechanisms and insight to physiological responses. *Acta Physiologica* 210(4):768-789.

IOM (Institute of Medicine). 1995. *Not eating enough: Overcoming underconsumption of military operational rations*. Washington, DC: National Academy Press.

IOM. 1999. *Committee on Military Nutrition Research: Activity report*. Washington, DC: National Academy Press.

IOM. 2006. *Dietary reference intakes: The essential guide to nutrient requirements*. Washington, DC: The National Academies Press.

IOM. 2008. *Review of NASA's human research evidence books: A letter report.* Washington, DC: The National Academies Press.

IOM. 2011. *Finding what works in health care: Standards for systematic reviews.* Washington, DC: The National Academies Press.

IOM. 2014. *Review of NASA's evidence reports on human health risks: 2013 letter report.* Washington, DC: The National Academies Press.

IOM. 2015. *Review of NASA's evidence reports on human health risks: 2014 letter report.* Washington, DC: The National Academies Press.

Jersey, S. L., R. A. Jesinger, and P. Palka. 2013. Brain magnetic resonance imaging anomalies in U-2 pilots with neurological decompression sickness. *Aviation, Space, and Environmental Medicine* 84(1):3-11.

Jonas, W. B. and S. J. Montain. 2014. Nutritional armor: Omega-3 for the warfighter. In *Military Medicine: International Journal of AMSUS* 179(11). http://publications.amsus.org/pb/assets/raw/Supplements/179_11_Supplement.pdf (accessed November 20, 2015).

Josephson, E. S. 2015. Advantages, problems, and experiences of irradiated foods. http://history.nasa.gov/SP-202/sess2.5.htm (accessed November 11, 2015).

Landon, L. B., W. B. Vessey, and J. D. Barrett. 2015. *Risk of performance and behavioral health decrements due to inadequate cooperation, coordination, communication, and psychosocial adaptation within a team.* https://humanresearchroadmap.nasa.gov/evidence/reports/Team.pdf (accessed November 17, 2015).

Lee, S. M., A. D. Moore, M. E. Everett, M. B. Stenger, and S. H. Platts. 2010. Aerobic exercise deconditioning and countermeasures during bed rest. *Aviation, Space, and Environmental Medicine* 81(1):52-63.

Ley, W., and W. Von Braun. 1956. *The exploration of Mars.* London: Sidgwick & Jackson.

Mahon, R., D. Klaus, T. Neuman, A. Pilmanis, and D. Regis. 2014. *Decompression sickness/extravehicular activity risks standing review panel.* http://ntrs.nasa.gov/archive/nasa/casi.ntrs.nasa.gov/20150008160.pdf (accessed October 2, 2015).

McGuire, S., P. Sherman, L. Profenna, P. Grogan, J. Sladky, A. Brown, A. Robinson, L. Rowland, E. Hong, B. Patel, D. Tate, E. S. Kawano, P. Fox, and P. Kochunov. 2013. White matter hyperintensities on MRI in high-altitude U-2 pilots. *Neurology* 81(8):729-735.

McManus, K., L. Antinoro, and F. Sacks. 2001. A randomized controlled trial of a moderate-fat, low-energy diet compared with a low fat, low-energy diet for weight loss in overweight adults. *International Journal of Obesity and Related Metabolic Disorders* 25(10):1503-1511.

Mekjavic, I. B., S. N. Kounalakis, M. E. Keramidas, G. Biolo, M. Narici, and O. Eiken. 2012. Heat production and heat loss responses to cold water immersion after 35 days horizontal bed rest. *Aviation, Space, and Environmental Medicine* 83(5):472-476.

NASA (National Aeronautics and Space Administration). 2013a. *Evidence book overview.* http://humanresearchroadmap.nasa.gov/Evidence/#overview (accessed November 30, 2014).

NASA. 2013b. *Human Research Program, Revision F.* http://www.nasa.gov/pdf/579466main_Human_Research_Program_Requirements_DocumentRevF.pdf (accessed November 17, 2014).

NASA. 2014a. *Human research roadmap: Introduction.* http://humanresearchroadmap.nasa.gov/intro (accessed September 30, 2015).

NASA. 2014b. The NASA Z-2 suit: Spacesuit design vote. https://jscfeatures.jsc.nasa.gov/z2 (accessed November 18, 2015).

NASA. 2015. *Risk of injury and compromised performance due to EVA operations.* http://humanresearchroadmap.nasa.gov/Risks/risk.aspx?i=84 (accessed October 19, 2015).

Newman, D. J., J. Hoffman, K. Bethke, C. Carr, N. Jordan, L. Sim, N. Campos, C. Conlee, B. Smith, J. Wilcox, G. Trotti, and MIDE-Technologies. 2005. *Astronaut bio-suit system for exploration class missions.* http://www.niac.usra.edu/files/studies/final_report/833Newman.pdf (accessed October 2, 2015).

Pedersen, B. K., and M. A. Febbraio. 2012. Muscles, exercise and obesity: Skeletal muscle as a secretory organ. *Nature Reviews. Endocrinology* 8(8):457-465.

Perchonok, M., D. Barta, M. Lawson, J. Joshi, and D. Russo. 2003. *Advanced food technology workshop report: Volume 1.* https://www.nasa.gov/centers/johnson/pdf/486020main_AdvFoodTechReportVol1.pdf (accessed November 11, 2015).

Perchonok, M., G. Douglas, and M. Cooper. 2012. *NASA evidence report: Risk of performance decrement and crew illness due to an inadequate food system.* http://humanresearchroadmap.nasa.gov/evidence/reports/Food.pdf (accessed September 29, 2015).

Pilmanis, A. A., J. T. Webb, U. I. Balldin, J. Conkin, and J. R. Fischer. 2010. Air break during preoxygenation and risk of altitude decompression sickness. *Aviation, Space, and Environmental Medicine* 81(10):944-950.

Ploutz-Snyder, L., S. Bloomfield, S. M. Smith, S. K. Hunter, K. Templeton, and D. Bemben. 2014. Effects of sex and gender on adaptation to space: Musculoskeletal health. *Journal of Women's Health* 23(11):963-966.

Ploutz-Snyder, L., J. Ryder, K. English, F. Haddad, and K. Baldwin. 2015. *NASA evidence report: Risk of impaired performance due to reduced muscle mass, strength, and endurance.* http://humanresearchroadmap.nasa.gov/evidence/reports/Muscle.pdf (accessed September 29, 2015).

Pratesi, A., F. Tarantini, and M. Di Bari. 2013. Skeletal muscle: An endocrine organ. *Clinical Cases in Mineral and Bone Metabolism* 10(1):11-14.

Reisner, A. T., D. Xu, K. L. Ryan, V. A. Convertino, C. A. Rickards, and R. Mukkamala. 2011. Monitoring non-invasive cardiac output and stroke volume during experimental human hypovolaemia and resuscitation. *British Journal of Anaesthesia* 106(1):23-30.

Ricci, F., R. De Caterina, and A. Fedorowski. 2015. Orthostatic hypotension: Epidemiology, prognosis, and treatment. *Journal of the American College of Cardiology* 66(7):848-860.

Sándor, A., S. V. Schuh, and B. F. Gore. 2013. *NASA evidence report: Risk of inadequate critical task design.* https://humanresearchroadmap.nasa.gov/evidence/reports/TASK.pdf (accessed October 2, 2015).

Scheuring, R. A., J. A. Jones, J. D. Polk, D. B. Gillis, J. Schmid, J. M. Duncan, J. R. Davis, and J. D. Novak. 2007. *The Apollo Medical Operations Project: Recommendations to improve crew health and performance for future exploration missions and lunar surface operations*. NASA/TM-2007-214755. http://ntrs.nasa.gov/archive/nasa/casi.ntrs.nasa.gov/20070030109.pdf (accessed September 29, 2015).

Sekhon, B. S. 2010. Food nanotechnology: An overview. *Journal of Nanotechnology, Science and Applications* 3:1-15.

Smith, S. M., S. R. Zwart, and M. Heer. 2015. *NASA evidence report: Risk factor of inadequate nutrition.* http://humanresearchroadmap.nasa.gov/evidence/reports/Nutrition-20150105.pdf?rnd=0.506950985410694 (accessed September 4, 2015).

Stabley, J. N., J. M. Dominguez II, C. E. Dominguez, F. R. Mora Solis, J. Ahlgren, B. J. Behnke, J. M. Muller-Delp, and M. D. Delp. 2012. Spaceflight reduces vasoconstrictor responsiveness of skeletal muscle resistance arteries in mice. *Journal of Applied Physiology* 113(9):1439-1445.

Steinberg, S., R. Mahon, D. Klaus, T. Neuman, A. Pilmanis, and D. Regis. 2014. *2014 Decompression sickness/extravehicular activity risks standing review panel.* NASA Technical Report JSC-CN-33307. http://ntrs.nasa.gov/archive/nasa/casi.ntrs.nasa.gov/20150008159.pdf (accessed September 30, 2015).

Stenger, M., S. H. Platts, S. M. C. Lee, C. M. Westby, T. R. Phillips, N. M. Arzeno, S. Johnston, and L. Mulugeta. 2015. *NASA evidence report: Risk of orthostatic intolerance during re-exposure to gravity.* http://humanresearchroadmap.nasa.gov/evidence/reports/ORTHO.pdf (accessed September 29, 2015).

Stuster, J. 2010. Acceptable risk: The human mission to Mars. *Journal of Cosmology* 12:3566-3577.

Taylor, C. R., M. Hanna, B. J. Behnke, J. N. Stabley, D. J. McCullough, R. T. Davis III, P. Ghosh, A. Papadopoulos, J. M. Muller-Delp, and M. D. Delp. 2013. Spaceflight-induced alterations in cerebral artery vasoconstrictor, mechanical, and structural properties: Implications for elevated cerebral perfusion and intracranial pressure. *The FASEB Journal* 27(6):2282-2292.

Trappe, T. A., F. White, C. P. Lambert, D. Cesar, M. Hellerstein, and W. J. Evans. 2002. Effect of ibuprofen and acetaminophen on postexercise muscle protein synthesis. *American Journal of Physiology: Endocrinology and Metabolism* 282(3):E551-E556.

Trappe, T. A., C. C. Carroll, J. M. Dickinson, J. K. LeMoine, J. M. Haus, B. E. Sullivan, J. D. Lee, B. Jemiolo, E. M. Weinheimer, and C. J. Hollon. 2011. Influence of acetaminophen and ibuprofen on skeletal muscle adaptations to resistance exercise in older adults. *American Journal of Physiology: Regulatory, Integrative and Comparative Physiology* 300(3):R655-R662.

USDA/HHS (U.S. Department of Agriculture and U.S. Department of Health and Human Services). 2015. *Scientific report of the 2015 Dietary Guidelines Advisory Committee.* http://health.gov/dietaryguidelines/2015-scientific-report/PDFs/Scientific-Report-of-the-2015-Dietary-Guidelines-Advisory-Committee.pdf (accessed November 13, 2015).

Waldie, J. M. A. 2005. *Mechanical counter pressure space suits: Advantages, limitations, and concepts for Martian exploration.* Lakewood, CO: The Mars Society.

Wallace, B. C., I. J. Dahabreh, C. H. Schmid, J. Lau, and T. A. Trikalinos. 2013. Modernizing the systematic review process to inform comparative effectiveness: Tools and methods. *Journal of Comparative Effectiveness Research* 2(3):273-282.

Wallace, J. P., G. T. Trail, and W. D. Franke. 2010. LBNP tolerance analyzed retrospectively using a structural equation model. *Aviation, Space, and Environmental Medicine* 81(4):363-368.

Webb, P. 1968. The space activity suit: An elastic leotard for extravehicular activity. *Aerospace Medicine* 39:376-383.

Webb, P., and J. Annis. 1967. *The principle of the space activity suit.* Washington, DC: NASA.

Zeizel, S. H., and M. A. Caudill. 2010. Choline. *Advances in Nutrition* 1:46-48.

Zeizel, S. H., and K. D. Corbin. 2012. Choline. In *Present knowledge in nutrition*, 10th ed., edited by J. W. Erdman, Jr., I. A. MacDonald, and S. H. Zeisel. Oxford, UK: Wiley-Blackwell.

Zeizel, S. H., and K. A. da Costa. 2009. Choline: An essential nutrient in public health. *Nutrition Reviews* 67(11):616-623.

Zeizel, S. H., M. H. Mar, J. C. Howe, and J. M. Holden. 2003. Concentrations of choline-containing compounds and betaine in common foods. *The Journal of Nutrition* 133(5):1302-1307.

A

Meeting Agendas

First Meeting of the
2015 Committee to Review NASA's Evidence Reports
on Human Health Risks

Web Conference

May 4, 2015

OPEN SESSION

12:00 – 12:05 p.m.	**Welcome and Opening Remarks** *Carol Scott-Conner, Committee Chair*
12:05 – 12:45 p.m.	**Official Committee Charge and Discussion of First and Second Letter Reports** *Mark Shelhamer, Chief Scientist, Human Research Program, NASA* **Discussion of Statement of Task and 2015 Reports with the Committee** *Facilitator: Carol Scott-Conner, Committee Chair*
12:45 p.m.	**Adjourn Open Session**

Second Meeting of the
2015 Committee to Review NASA's Evidence Reports
on Human Health Risks

Keck Center of the National Academies
500 Fifth Street, NW, Room 101
Washington, DC

June 22-23, 2015
Keck 101

OPEN SESSION

June 22, 2015

9:00 – 9:15 a.m.	**Welcome** *Carol Scott-Conner, Committee Chair*

9:15 – 10:45 a.m.	**Panel 1: EVA and DCS**
	
	• *Risk of Compromised EVA Performance and Crew Health Due to Inadequate EVA Suit Systems*
	• *DCS – Risk of Decompression Sickness*
	
	Facilitator: Jack Stuster
	
	9:15 – 10:15 Presentations
	• EVA
	  o Michael Lopez-Alegria, MLA Space LLC (*via WebEx*)
	• Decompression Sickness
	  o Neal Pollock, Duke University
	
	10:15 – 10:45 Discussion with the Committee

10:45 – 11:00 a.m.	**BREAK**

11:00 a.m. – 12:30 p.m. **Panel 2: Orthostatic, Aerobic, and Muscle**

- *Ortho – Risk of Orthostatic Intolerance During Re-exposure to Gravity*
- *Aerobic – Risk of Reduced Physical Performance Capabilities Due to Reduced Aerobic Capacity*
- *Muscle – Risk of Impaired Performance Due to Reduced Muscle Mass, Strength, and Endurance*

Facilitator: Jim Pawelczyk

11:00 – 12:00 Presentations

- Aerobic
  - Ben Levine, University of Texas Southwestern (*Attending via WebEx*)
- Muscle
  - Bob Fitts, Marquette University (*Attending*)
- Orthostatic Intolerance
  - Victor Convertino, U.S. Army Institute of Surgical Research (*Attending via WebEx*)

12:00 – 12:30 Discussion with the Committee

12:30 – 1:15 p.m. **Lunch - Keck Atrium**
(Committee members and speakers have blue lunch tickets – please sign the ticket and turn it in to the cashier)

1:15 – 2:30 p.m. **Panel 3: Food and Nutrition**

- *Risk of Performance Decrement and Crew Illness Due to an Inadequate Food System*
- *Nutrition – Risk Factor of Inadequate Nutrition*

Facilitator: Dan Masys

1:15 – 2:15 Presentations

- Scott Montain and Betty Davis, U.S. Army (*Attending via WebEx*)
- Alice Lichtenstein, Tufts University
- Nancy Turner, Texas A&M University (*Attending via WebEx*)

2:15 – 2:30 Discussion with the Committee

2:30 – 2:45 p.m. **BREAK**

2:45 – 4:00 p.m. **Discussion–Interactions of Risks**

4:00 – 4:20 p.m. **Public Comment**

4:20 – 4:30 p.m. **Closing Remarks**
Dan Masys, Committee Vice Chair

B

Committee Biographical Sketches

Carol E. H. Scott-Conner, M.D., Ph.D., M.B.A. (*Chair*), is professor emeritus in the Department of Surgery, University of Iowa, Iowa City. Dr. Scott-Conner received her undergraduate training in electrical engineering from the Massachusetts Institute of Technology and worked as an engineer before attending medical school at New York University (NYU). In 1976, she received her M.D. from NYU, where she also completed a residency in surgery. After leaving NYU, she joined the faculty at Marshall University and then moved to the University of Mississippi. During her tenure there, she earned a Ph.D. in anatomy from the University of Kentucky and an M.B.A. In 1995, she became professor and head of surgery at the University of Iowa. Dr. Scott-Conner has been active on 22 editorial boards and has written more than 200 original papers, abstracts, reviews, and book chapters. She is certified by the National Board of Medical Examiners and the American Board of Surgery and has a certification of added qualifications in surgical critical care. Dr. Scott-Conner has served on a number of Institute of Medicine committees, and she chairs the National Academies of Sciences, Engineering and Medicine Standing Committee on Aerospace Medicine and the Medicine of Extreme Environments.

Daniel R. Masys, M.D. (*Vice Chair*), is an affiliate professor of biomedical and health informatics at the University of Washington School of Medicine, where he joined the Department of Biomedical Informatics and Medical Education in 2011. Previously, he served as a professor and the chair of the Department of Biomedical Informatics and a professor of medicine at the Vanderbilt University School of Medicine. An honors graduate of Princeton University and the Ohio State University College of

Medicine, he completed postgraduate training in internal medicine, hematology, and medical oncology at the University of California, San Diego (UCSD), and the Naval Regional Medical Center, San Diego. He served as chief of the International Cancer Research Data Bank of the National Cancer Institute, National Institutes of Health, and was director of the Lister Hill National Center for Biomedical Communications, which is the computer research and development division of the National Library of Medicine. He also served as director of biomedical informatics at the UCSD School of Medicine, director of the UCSD Human Research Protections Program, and professor of medicine. Dr. Masys is an elected member of the National Academy of Medicine (NAM). He is a diplomate of the American Board of Internal Medicine in medicine, hematology, and medical oncology. He is a fellow of the American College of Physicians and fellow and past president of the American College of Medical Informatics. Dr. Masys served as a member of the Institute of Medicine (IOM) Committee on Aerospace Medicine and the Medicine of Extreme Environments and chaired the 2008 IOM review of NASA's Human Research Program evidence books.

Susan A. Bloomfield, Ph.D., earned her B.S. in biology at Oberlin College (Ohio) and her M.A. in physical education (exercise physiology) at the University of Iowa. After completing a Ph.D. (exercise physiology) at Ohio State University, Dr. Bloomfield joined the faculty in the Department of Health and Kinesiology at Texas A&M University in 1993, where she currently holds the rank of professor and is director of the Bone Biology Laboratory. In addition, she serves as assistant provost in the Texas A&M Office of Graduate and Professional Studies. Her research interests focus on the integrative physiology of bone, with specific reference to adaptations to disuse, microgravity, and caloric deficiency and how the sympathetic nervous system, altered blood flow, and endocrine factors modify those adaptations. Her more recent work has focused on the independent and combined effects of partial weight bearing and simulated space radiation on the integrity of bone and muscle, involving several experiments at Brookhaven National Laboratory. Collaborations with muscle biologists have enabled definition of concurrent changes in muscle–bone pairs with disuse and/or radiation exposure. Her work has been funded by the National Space Biomedical Research Institute (NSBRI), the U.S. Department of Defense, and, currently, NASA's Space

Biology Program. From 2000 to 2012, Dr. Bloomfield served as the associate lead for the Bone Loss (later, Musculoskeletal Alterations) Team within the NSBRI, and she has served on numerous NASA and European Space Agency review panels during the past 14 years. She is a member of the Texas A&M Department of Nutrition and Food Sciences graduate faculty and is an associate member of the Texas A&M University Health Sciences Center School of Graduate Studies.

C. Patrick Dunne, Ph.D., has a Ph.D. in biochemistry from Brandeis University and a B.A. in chemistry from the University of California, Riverside. Before joining the U.S. Army Research Center in Natick, Massachusetts, in 1979, Dr. Dunne was on the faculty at the University of Detroit and California State University at Long Beach; he also was a postdoctoral associate in biochemistry at Michigan State University. Dr. Dunne retired as the Senior Advisor in Advanced Processing and Nutritional Biochemistry for the Department of Defense Combat Feeding Project of the U.S. Army Natick Soldier Center of the Soldier and Biological Chemical Command in September 2012. Since 1991 he was the project officer of the Cold Preservation Project at Natick and has taken a lead role in dual use science and technology projects in advanced food processing technologies—pulsed electric field, high pressure and microwave processing. His research efforts in food biochemistry and nutritional biochemistry supported the development of improved rations for the military. Dr. Dunne was a founding member of the new Nonthermal Processing Division of the Institute of Food Technologists (IFT); he was elected the first chair of that division in 1999. He was the IFT Solberg Award winner in 2005 for fostering collaborations among academia, industry, and government researchers. He was named an IFT Fellow in 2009 and was one of the team of five who were given the IFT 2010 Research and Development Award for the microwave sterilization process. In 2014 Dr. Dunne was named the recipient of the IFT's highest award, the Nicholas Appert Award; he was also awarded the Institute of Food Safety and Health Food Safety Award in 2011. Dr. Dunne maintains an active interest in science education; he was an elected member of the Framingham, Massachusetts, School Committee for 12 years.

Brad Holschuh, Ph.D., is an assistant professor of wearable technology and human factors at the University of Minnesota (UMN), and is co-director of the Wearable Technology Laboratory in the UMN College of Design. Dr. Holschuh earned his Ph.D. degree from the Department of

Aeronautics and Astronautics at the Massachusetts Institute of Technology (MIT), and was a member of the inaugural class of NASA Space Technology Research Fellows. As a graduate student and postdoctoral associate in the MIT Man-Vehicle Laboratory, Dr. Holschuh focused on active materials development for mechanical counter-pressure space suits in partnership with the NASA Johnson Space Center. Dr. Holschuh's current research focuses on topics related to wearable technologies to improve human performance both in space and on Earth. He is specifically interested in developing wearable smart systems using additive manufacturing, active materials, and onboard sensing and computing systems to address a variety of space, biomedical, military, and commercial challenges. His work encompasses wearable technology, aerospace engineering, materials science, human factors, textile engineering, and biomedical device development.

Michael J. Joyner, M.D., is a physician-researcher focused on human performance and exercise physiology. Using humans as his model system, he has made major contributions to understanding muscle and skin blood flow, blood pressure regulation, and human athletic performance. His ideas about human performance are widely quoted in both the popular media and scientific publications. Dr. Joyner has been a consultant to the National Institutes of Health (NIH) and NASA and has held leadership positions with prestigious scientific journals. His research lab at Mayo Clinic has been continuously funded by the NIH since 1993. Mayo Clinic named him a Distinguished Investigator in 2010. His lab has provided significant educational opportunities for students and trainees, many of whom have established independent research programs at leading institutions throughout the world. Both his undergraduate (1981) and medical (1987) degrees are from the University of Arizona. Dr. Joyner completed his residency and research training at Mayo Clinic, where he continues to practice anesthesiology, has held numerous leadership positions, and is the Frank R. and Shari Caywood Professor of Anesthesiology.

James A. Pawelczyk, Ph.D., is an associate professor of physiology, kinesiology, and medicine at Pennsylvania State University. Dr. Pawelczyk served as a payload specialist on STS-90 Neurolab (April 17 to May 3, 1998); the experiments on board the space shuttle *Columbia* flight focused on the effects of microgravity on the brain and nervous system. Dr. Pawelczyk is a former member of the NASA Life Sciences Advisory

Subcommittee in the Office of Biological and Physical Research, and he served as a member of NASA's ReMaP Task Force in 2002, which was charged with reprioritizing research on the space station. Dr. Pawelczyk's research areas include central neural control of the cardiovascular system and compensatory mechanisms to conditioning and deconditioning. He received his M.S. in physiology from Pennsylvania State University and his Ph.D. in biology (physiology) from the University of North Texas. He chaired the National Research Council (NRC) Decadal Survey on Biological and Physical Sciences in Space: Integrative and Translational Research for the Human System Panel and chaired an Institute of Medicine (IOM) report on NASA's directed research programs in 2012. He has served on several NRC and IOM committees and recently completed rotations on the National Academies of Sciences, Engineering, and Medicine Committee on Aerospace Medicine and the Medicine of Extreme Environments and the Academies Space Studies Board.

K. P. Sandeep, Ph.D., is Professor of Food Science in the College of Agriculture and Life Sciences at North Carolina State University. He received his doctorate from Pennsylvania State University. His primary research interests are in food engineering, specifically thermal/aseptic processing of particulate foods and various aspects of fluid mechanics and heat transfer.

Robert L. Satcher, Jr., M.D., Ph.D., is an assistant professor of surgical oncology at MD Anderson Cancer Center. He earned a Ph.D. in chemical engineering from the Massachusetts Institute of Technology in 1993 and an M.D. from Harvard Medical School in 1994. His medical specialties are orthopedics and oncology, and he has done much work in treating bone cancer in adults and children. Selected as an astronaut candidate by NASA in 2004, he completed his training 2 years later. He was aboard the space shuttle *Atlantis* that journeyed to the International Space Station for almost 11 days in November 2009. Classified as a mission specialist, he studied the influence of zero gravity on muscles and bone density as well as the effects of space on the immune system. He also used his surgical training to install an antenna and help repair two robotic arms on the space station. Dr. Satcher is director of the eHealth Research Institute at Texas Medical Center and a member of the User Panel at the National Space and Biomedical Research Institute (NSBRI). He is a frequent reviewer and adviser for medical issues related to spaceflight.

Jack Stuster, Ph.D., is the vice president and principal scientist of Anacapa Sciences, Inc., a human factors and applied behavioral sciences research firm. He received a bachelor's degree in experimental psychology from the University of California, Santa Barbara, and a master's and Ph.D. degrees in anthropology from the same institution. Dr. Stuster is a certified professional ergonomist, specializing in the measurement and enhancement of human performance in extreme environments. He has analyzed the tasks performed by U.S. Navy SEALs, SEAL delivery-vehicle pilots and navigators, explosive ordnance disposal technicians, crews of high-speed hovercraft, maintenance personnel, and military leaders. Dr. Stuster's work for NASA began in 1982 with a systems analysis of space shuttle refurbishing procedures, which has been followed by studies of conditions on Earth that are analogous to those found on space missions. Dr. Stuster has been awarded fellow status by the Human Factors and Ergonomics Society and the Borneo Research Society. He was a member of the Science Council of NASA's Institute for Advanced Concepts and is now a member of the External Advisory Council of the National Space Biomedical Research Institute. He has also served on several government advisory groups, including the standing committee of the National Academies of Sciences, Engineering, and Medicine's Board on Army Science and Technology to support the efforts of the Joint Improvised Explosive Device Defeat Organization, for which he received a patriotic Civilian Service Commendation in 2011. He currently serves as the principal investigator of the Journals Flight Experiment and of the development of the Cultural Depot, an information-sharing system for use by special operations personnel.

Scott Trappe, Ph.D., is the director of the Human Performance Laboratory and John and Janice Fisher Endowed Chair in Exercise Science at Ball State University. Dr. Trappe earned his undergraduate training at the University of Northern Iowa (1989). He worked for U.S. Swimming at the Olympic Training Center in Colorado Springs while conducting his graduate studies at the University of Colorado. His Ph.D. training was with Dr. David Costill at Ball State University (1994) and postdoctoral training in muscle physiology with Dr. Robert Fitts at Marquette University (1997). Dr. Trappe has been the principal investigator on several National Institutes of Health (NIH) and NASA human-based exercise physiology research projects. The aim of his research program is to connect biological and physiological measures at the cellular level with whole body outcomes in response to acute and chronic exercise perturbations. For much of his career, Dr. Trappe has been working with NASA to help optimize the exercise prescription for astronauts. He has conducted several exercise training studies in older adults, aging athletes, and various college and elite athletes. Dr. Trappe has served on several NIH study sections and NASA committees, including the 2008 Institute of Medicine report on NASA's human research program. He is a fellow of the American College of Sports Medicine and a member of the American Physiological Society.

Peter D. Wagner, M.D., is Distinguished Professor of Medicine & Bioengineering at the University of California, San Diego (UCSD), in La Jolla, California. After obtaining his M.B., B.S., and B.Sc. (Medicine) degrees from Sydney University in 1968, he did postdoctoral work with Professor John West at UCSD. He then joined the UCSD medical faculty and has remained there to the present time. His research addresses the theoretical and experimental basis of oxygen transport and its limitations in the lungs and skeletal muscles in health and disease. A particular focus is on muscle capillary growth regulation using molecular biological approaches in integrated systems. He has served as a National Institutes of Health (NIH) study section member and chair, associate editor of the *Journal of Clinical Investigation*, and associate editor of the *Journal of Applied Physiology*. He was president of the American Thoracic Society 2005-2006, and was president of the American Physiological Society 2010-2011. Current major responsibilities include serving as editor of the *Journal of Applied Physiology*, editor of two sections of Comprehensive Physiology, chair of an NIH study section, and treasurer of the International Union of Physiological Sciences. He has published more than 350 peer-reviewed research articles and more than 120 invited chapters and other contributions.

Gayle E. Woloschak, Ph.D., is a professor in the Department of Radiology at the Feinberg School of Medicine at Northwestern University. Her research interests include studies of the molecular biology of lymphocyte and motor neuron abnormalities in DNA repair–deficient mice, studies of radiation-inducible nanoparticles, and the analysis of molecular mechanisms of oncogenesis in radiation-induced tumors. She received her Ph.D. in medical sciences (microbiology) from the Medical College of Ohio and did postdoctoral training in the departments of immunology and molecular biology at the Mayo Clinic. Dr. Woloschak was a senior molecular biologist and group leader of the Biosciences Division at Argonne National Laboratory, and a senior fellow at the Nanosciences Consortium of Argonne National Laboratory–University of Chicago. She has served as a member on the National Institutes of Health's radiation study section and on the National Academies of Sciences, Engineering, and Medicine Committee on the Evaluation of Radiation Shielding for Space Exploration, and she has chaired NASA's peer-review radiation biology committee.

Laurence R. Young, Sc.D., is professor of astronautics and professor of health sciences and technology at the Massachusetts Institute of Technology (MIT). He was the founding director (1997-2001) of the National Space Biomedical Research Institute. Dr. Young is a full member of the International Academy of Astronautics. He received an A.B. from Amherst College; a certificate in applied mathematics from the Sorbonne in Paris, as a French government fellow; and S.B. and S.M. degrees in electrical engineering and an Sc.D. in instrumentation from MIT. He joined the MIT faculty in 1962 and co-founded the Man Vehicle Laboratory, which does research on the visual and vestibular systems, visual-vestibular interaction, flight simulation, space motion sickness, and manual control and displays. In 1991, Dr. Young was selected as a payload specialist for Spacelab Life Sciences 2. He spent 2 years in training at the Johnson Space Center and served as alternate payload specialist during the October 1993 mission. He was chairman of the Harvard–MIT Committee on Biomedical Engineering and Physics and the interdepartmental Ph.D. program in biomedical engineering, and he directs the Harvard–MIT Program in Bioastronautics. Dr. Young is a member of the National Academy of Medicine and the National Academy of Engineering and has served on many National Academies of Sciences, Engineering, and Medicine committees, including the Committee on Aerospace Medicine and the Medicine of Extreme Environments.